# Living Life As A Joyful Being

be ready for
whatever life brings!

By Joy Jangdhari

Blessings!
Joy Jangdhari

**Living Life As A Joyful Being:** *be ready for whatever life brings!*
 Published and distributed in the United States by Joy Jangdhari, P.O. Box 3752 New York, NY 10185-3752
www.JoyJangdhari.com



The author of this book does not dispense medical advice or prescribe the use of any techniques as a form of treatment for physical or medical problems. The intent of the author is only to offer information of a general nature to help you in your quest for emotional well being. In the event you use any of the information in this book for yourself, which is your constitutional right, the author and the publisher assume no responsibility for your actions.

ISBN: 978-0-615-43289-2

FOURTH EDITION

I dedicate this book to all

*Joyful Beings...*

Past,
Present
&
Future

# Notes

# Contents


preface ........................................ ix

introduction ........................................ 1

chapter 1 – looking within ........................................ 5

chapter 2 – lights, camera, action ........................................ 15

chapter 3 – bringing awareness ........................................ 23

chapter 4 – staying in the present moment ........................................ 29

chapter 5 – calming the mind ........................................ 41

chapter 6 – letting go ........................................ 48

chapter 7 – when buttons are pushed ........................................ 59

chapter 8 – climbing the emotional hill ........................................ 73

chapter 9 – treating yourself with kindness ........................................ 79

chapter 10 – mechanics of the mind ........................................ 87

chapter 11 – integrity with yourself ........................................ 92

chapter 12 – introspection ........................................ 99

chapter 13 – visualization ........................................ 105

chapter 14 – a few good moves ........................................ 112

chapter 15 – joyful being ........................................ 114

# Notes

# Preface

Who wouldn't like a joyful life? And a "guide" to get there? Why…yes please! Begin your reading of my guide to living life as a joyful being in that spirit…enjoy! Take a little or take a lot, but have fun! Each step is meant to lighten your emotional load. This is not a heavy-weighted philosophy, but a study of possibilities. And one thing the reader can add to this book to transform any hint of philosophy into a real life experience is…

***Action***.

Many of my readers are blessed with fulfilling and contented lives. They will read this book to "compare notes", enjoying the shared thoughts as well as the contrasts.

**This book, for them, will be a gallery of perspective**.

Some readers have lives that function, and include happiness, as well as frustrations, but have always felt there was some small part of their mind, heart, or soul that was missing. They felt something was needed for them to feel more peaceful, satisfied, or complete, and they have a desire to study and expand themselves to their full potentials.

**This book, for them, will be a tool**.

However, there are readers who remain in my prayers, and could benefit from all of our prayers. They are those who suffer in the dark with disappointments that follow closely behind what happiness they find. They react, then react again to that reaction, and react again, until their lives feel like a pinball machine. By whatever circumstances those persons have found this book in front of them, it is my hope that it is with the will to make life better.

**This book, for them, is a Guide**.

And it is for them that I write this book.

Be Ready for Whatever Life Brings.

**And with you, bring Love, Patience, and Clarity.**

**- Joy Jangdhari**

# Introduction

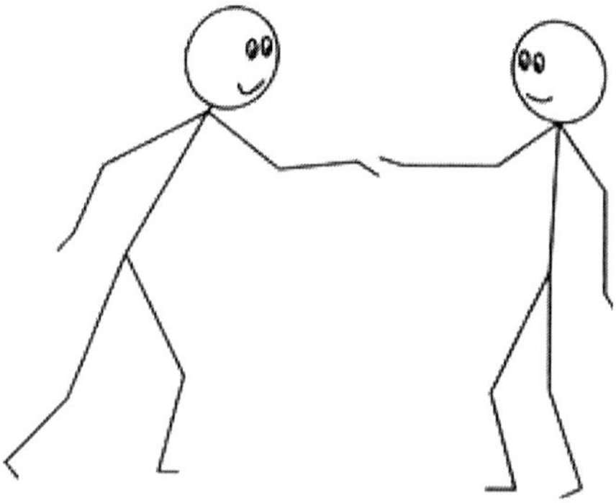

Welcome all! You are about to take a journey to explore new (and old!) paths, discover fresh perspectives, and create possibilities. Through self-study you will look at any beliefs, fears, reactions and desires that limit you and prevent you from living fully, authentically, and joyfully. Through regular practice you will open doors to look within at the many different facets of your life. You will uncover "masks" you made for yourself to protect yourself and survive in this world. You will create the awareness and balance of a clear and understanding mind.

In your practice, by using breath work you will deepen your awareness of your thoughts, words, and actions. You will learn to let go of the past, begin to release what you no longer need, and plant the seeds of new experiences. Through this process you will gain the courage, aliveness, and creativity to touch, move and inspire yourself and others.

As you leave the old mechanical habits behind, you will become more conscious and aware, and you will feel the release of tension from your body. Feeling "at home" within yourself, you will experience peace, unity, and deep joy. You will be in touch with that place inside yourself where YOU are a *Joyful Being*!

Throughout this book there are small stories or metaphors included to provide examples of what is being discussed. However, remember each person uniquely maps his or her own journey. It is up to you to determine where these concepts fit in your life. This book can be your resource, your guide, and your tool for *your* unique journey. Take from it what you will, and know that you are not alone.

## Being

*It is the letting go of all the*
*Should's, the must's, the have-to's,*
*The have-nots, the cannot's*
*The doubts and the guilt.*

*It is allowing your thoughts to come forth-*
*Without judgment.*

*It is allowing yourself to feel-*
*Without judgment.*

*It is allowing yourself to be who you are-*
*Without judgment.*

*It is allowing yourself to do what you want-*
*Without judgment.*

*When you allow yourself to be,*
*You find*
*Peace, Freedom, Love and Joy*
*Within you.*

*(Author Unknown)*

# Chapter 1 - looking within

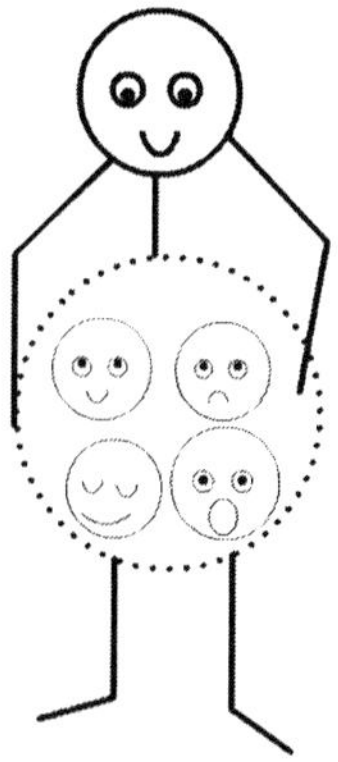

Have you ever driven somewhere you really wanted to go but had never been before? How did you know how to get there? Most likely you used some kind of map. Whether it was a map on paper or on the internet, you found your destination by looking for the address or town and said to yourself "that is where I want to be".

But was that all it took? No. You then had to find the location you were starting your trip from on the map as well (your home, the home of the friend you were picking up on the way, etc.) and decide on the best route to take to get from your starting point to your end point. Even if you asked someone else for directions, they would first have to know where you were coming from.

"Oh, but what about my GPS navigation system, where I only have to tell it where I want to go and it directs me!" you may say. True, but before that GPS navigation system can tell you which road to take, it first must figure out for itself where it, and you, are at that moment. There is no way around it. The only way to determine the best path to take is to know both where you want to end up and where you are now.

The same thing is true for this journey called life. You may know exactly where you want your life to lead, what qualities you want in your life, and the types of people and experiences you want to surround you. But until you take a look at your current situation (location) it will be very hard to know the best way to get to "the life of your dreams". The process of determining where you truly are "now" begins by looking within.

### *But it's dark and scary in there!*

Many of us have spent most of our lives avoiding that look within. We deny, repress, and suppress our feelings and pain of the past. We distract ourselves with work, play, sex, alcohol, drugs, food, shopping, watching hours and hours of television, surfing the internet, stressing about money, getting caught up in gossip (drama!) about who said and did what to whom, and much, much more.

While most of these activities can be fun, and some may even be healthy in balance (no, I'm not asking you to give up your favorite TV shows!) it is important to look at the context of WHY you are doing what you do. Is it because it is what you really want to be doing? Or is it because you are keeping busy or numbing yourself in an attempt to ignore what is really happening either in your life or in your head?

Let's take this one step at a time. If you are not ready to look within (and if you are not, that is fine...that is where you are...no judgments here!) then how about taking a look around? Take the time today to look at things that you do not normally notice. Notice the details of things. Enjoy the scenery, but look behind the scenes. Feel the open space around you.

Look at an object of your choosing like a photographer or an artist would look at it. Appreciate its beauty and the experience of seeing it. Give it your full attention for as long as you like. Examine the details, the colors, and the shapes. Look at it long enough to remember it later. Feel an appreciation for this opportunity to see something in a new way, and congratulate yourself for being open-minded enough to try.

Take a long look at something you find beautiful in nature: a sunrise, a flower, a landscape, or a shadow from a tree. Find something breathtaking. Look for rainbows. Feel an intimacy with your awakening awareness, the changing nature of your surroundings, and your unique perspective. By all means stop and smell the roses!

As you start to look more closely at the world around you, notice what you have been missing. You will find that you are witnessing some very uncommon and unique events. Looking at the night sky, you see a shooting star. The rising sun serves as the background for a group of migrating birds. Events are happening right in front of you that you may be missing because of distractions.

Determine how much time you spend indoors and how much time you spend outside. Feel the grass on your bare feet. Don't be afraid to walk on rocks. Do as much of this as you can. While you are outside, in the sun or under the clouds, in a city or in the country, go out and find something in nature that you may be taking for granted.

Being more aware of your surroundings enriches your life. By the end of the day, if you have found one thing that you enjoyed noticing, then you are on your way to being able to create extraordinary experiences. Then, when you are ready, you can begin using your new observational skills to begin looking at something truly beautiful and breathtaking...***YOU***.

Looking within is stepping into an internal realm. You become a witness to your own acts. Every category of self-investigation in this book has techniques to assist in creating internal balance. You will look at what emotions are "stuck" and trace the feelings back to the original event where you made a "stand" about who you were or what life was about. You will see rationalizations, justifications or even excuses as to why you have taken those stands.

The word "stand" seems to indicate an immovable, unchangeable position. But by looking within, you will find your "stands" are simply patterns of reactions and behaviors you took on based on past situations or experiences, and therefore completely within your power to change when the time is right for you.

Looking within is an act of integrity with yourself. It allows those patterns of reactions and behaviors to take a rest long enough to look one step deeper...to your thoughts and feelings at the moment of the incident. What were you thinking and feeling right before you reacted? Be still. Be quiet. Breathe evenly. Bring up in your mind the event that you feel has captured and held hostage your thoughts and feelings. Now surrender those thoughts and feelings to "your kidnappers".

Your "kidnappers" could be a person, event, situation, or justification in your mind. Temporarily surrender those stuck thoughts and feelings to whoever or whatever prompted your reaction. Allow your cycle of reaction and justification to slow and stop by simply observing it.

Looking within is a practice. The more you practice the farther back you can go, step by step. You can begin breaking the cycles of your own reactions, justifications and "stuck mind". Soon you will see a place where you are free to act on your own will, as your own joyful being.

Take a moment and check in with yourself, objectively observing each and every aspect of your life as if you were simply watching it all on a TV or movie screen. How do you see the situations in your life today? Are you seeing your "today" as an opportunity to have adventures and learn lessons, or just living life as a series of reactions based on memories and beliefs formed by the difficulties you encountered growing up? How do you see the world around you?

As you go through your life you usually look at other people and events from your own perspective and only see things and situations from your own point of view. Each and every one of us fights to defend and protect our own point of view and perspectives...but do you really know what you are fighting to defend and protect?

Where does your perspective come from? Your individual perspective depends on how you were raised, the events you experienced throughout your life, and the stories you told yourself about those events. Family, friends and peers, teachers, religious groups, cultural groups, etc., have taught you what was right, wrong, good, bad, acceptable, and unacceptable. This education in "who we should be" has been called "domestic conditioning" by some.

Much of the drama and distress in your life stems from not just your experiences, but the reactions, perceptions, beliefs and conditioning about those experiences that you have taken on from others.

Whether that information you received was a real truth, a distortion of the truth as presented by your parents, peers, or teachers, or stands that you took about yourself and your life, it lives in your mind as an image and a real condition. That image is not really you. It has a life of its own within you, until you examine it with objectivity and awareness to determine if the image is really your truth or one you have taken on from others.

Remember, we were once taught, and believed, that the world was flat. Now we know differently. The shift came when one person was courageous enough to say "hey, maybe we need to look at this belief and see if it is even really true!"

Each person's perspective is different. Each person has their own set of actions and reactions based on their experiences in the past. That is why you cannot take anything personally that is expressed to you by another person, and you do not always have to take on other people's perspectives as your own.

> **Example**: *The farmer likes, and needs, the rain for his field of vegetables. A racecar driver views the rain as dangerous during his time on the racetrack. Each person has a different reaction to the same event of rain, based on their individual perspective. Each man's success will depend on what he says to himself about the event and how this shifts his perspective. When we talk about a shifting of perspective, we are simply describing how a person changes his beliefs.*

Your thoughts are the author of the "stories" you have written about who you are and your experiences in life. Your stories are more fiction than reality until you look at your beliefs. Your stories try to live your life for you, and resist your taking control and really "deciding" what is *YOUR* truth. But the stories were not there when you first breathed life. As a baby your mind was completely open to everything around you.

Your concepts of right and wrong were not yet formed and the only self-image you had was your reflection in a mirror. As you grew up, your image of yourself became less based on your actual reflection (your own feelings and belief in yourself) and more based on the way other people saw you and convinced you they were seeing the "real you". As these images piled on over time, your self-image became more distorted.

If your mind was filled with negative comments, you will see yourself in a negative way. If you were given positive feedback, you will react in a more positive way to the world around you. You can become "addicted" to the opinions of others, slowly becoming less dependent on your ability to decide "who you are" for yourself and more dependent on the concept of "you" formed by others.

Step back from your own perspective and observe a situation objectively from the outside. This is a conscious action you have the option to take, so as not to get caught up in judgments, "stories", and reactions. In later chapters you will learn some techniques to write out your reactions after an upsetting event, question your beliefs, and dispute any irrational ideas. This will help you shift your perceptions in different life areas and see the truth about you and your life in a clear, more exciting way.

Only when we can identify our thoughts can we understand where they come from and how well they serve us. By bringing objectivity and awareness to our thoughts as they appear, we can evaluate the merit, worthiness and character of that thought. We can ask ourselves:

1. Who is the thinker of the thought? (Whose "tapes" am I playing...mom? dad? church? friend? etc.)
2. What is the purpose of this thought? (What feeling or emotion does it bring up for me?)
3. What will the consequences of this thought be? (Healthy or unhealthy habits being formed, judgmental/critical or positive/affirming messages to myself?)

This exercise will help you to train your mind to utilize its capacity to respond in a healthy way rather than a habitual way. This is one of the steps to emotional freedom.

### *When the look inward brings "bad news"*

You also know that when you begin to look within, there are usually some unpleasant feelings to confront. Many decisions and attitudes have developed in response to "negative conditioning" or "survival skills".

Not every lesson of your conditioning was based on accuracy or truth. Not every lesson that was valid in the past applies usefully to you now. What do you do with this information? The terrific part of this is that through awareness, you can begin creating new possibilities. Awareness means opening your eyes to see the truth, so you are no longer blind. Once you have confronted and recognized that past events have affected you, but do not permanently own you, then your perspective, your beliefs and the way you look inward changes forever. Just the act of becoming aware automatically allows a shift to begin.

# Chapter 2 - lights, camera, action

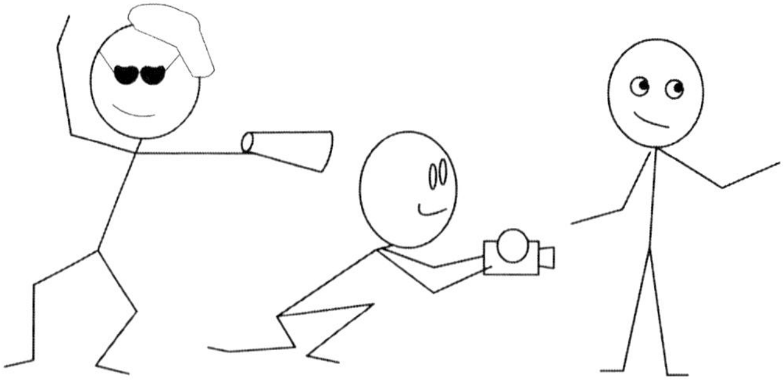

**"All the world's a stage,**

**and all the men and women merely players..."**

- *William Shakespeare*

You are always and all at once the actor, the scriptwriter, and the audience of your own life. You are also the camera operator, the director, and the critic. As actor you play the starring role, not in the sense of pretending, although you play many roles in your life.

You are the main character in your own TV show. You move about in the context of your surroundings, and according to social convention. You have an influence on what is happening. People and things around you may be affected by your words and actions. In return, you may be affected by the words and actions of others, either directly or indirectly. Because your words and actions are often a direct outcome of your thoughts, by altering your thoughts, words and actions you can re-write the script and completely change the plot of your show.

Today, as you walk into a store, a church, a bar, a school, a hospital, a bank, an office, a factory, or a field, what happens? Where do you go next? What do you do there? From scene, to scene, to scene, your life unfolds. Do you go from place to place, as a result of a conscious decision and choices you make? Or are your actions directed by others, by peer pressure, by popularity, or unconscious habit? Are you dragging your feet as you go to the next place, or are you running in joyous anticipation? Are the people you meet glad to see you, or not? The answer is a little of both, perhaps.

Your TV show is non-fiction. It is narrated in the first person voice, by you. There is no intermission, no commercial breaks. It has a beginning and an end. You cannot simply turn off the television when you no longer want to participate. It is performed live. You cannot edit out mistakes, but you can make corrections later. And you get to keep a recording, whether you like it or not. Your body is the actor and always in "live" mode. If you touch fire, you get burned. If you are in water, you get wet. If you are hit, you will bruise. If you are cut, you will bleed. You will feel both pleasant and unpleasant sensations.

But is there more to it than that? Yes. You are also the audience, the observer of your life, including your thoughts, words, actions and experiences. You have the ability to see yourself from an outside point-of-view. You can look in the mirror and see your physical body, and you can look inside and "see" your thoughts, beliefs, and even your dreams. You have the ability to be self-aware. You can only truly be the observer of your life when you see your life in a detached way, without the emotional "charge" that may linger from past experiences or worries and fears about future events. You are always the actor in your body, and the body is never in the past or future.

This is the point of reminding yourself to stay present. Sometimes you bang your knee on the table, or hit the car behind you in the parking lot, because you are too much in your mind, too much in the past or the future, to the point of distraction. Being too much in the past, the future, or other places removes your attention away from the immediacy of what is going on right now. As a result, "accidents" may happen that painfully bring us back to the present.

As the camera operator, you have the choice of what to zoom in on in your life. Where you focus your attention is completely up to you. Once you have experienced something, you can exaggerate it and make it something very large and important, or you can minimize it, blur it, fade it out, or delete it. This ability comes in very handy if you know how to use it to your advantage. *Become aware of what you focus on in your life.* Do you look for proof that life is hard, or do you choose to see the beauty in life? Do you look around, on guard, waiting for the next event to happen to you, or do you seek out people, places, and things that inspire you? Do you just go through each day feeling both empty and overwhelmed with no end in sight, or do you feel a sense of wonder, curiosity, and joy?

The more you develop your awareness skills, the more things you will notice, and the more present, connected and intuitive you will become. Increasing your self-awareness is not just about stopping to smell the roses, but about becoming more effective at adapting to changing circumstances and recognizing new opportunities and possibilities for your life.

As director of your life, you are responsible for your current situation. Where do you live? What language do you speak? Are you in a job you love, or just working to pay the bills? Do you see your life as a pleasure cruise, or do you feel like you are on a sinking ship? What type of education do you have? Do you have a lot of money? How much money do you owe? Are you healthy? Do you exercise? What do you like to eat? Do you have friends, co-workers, peers, family members, enemies? Who are they? Are you loved? Are you hated? Do you love? Do you hate? How do you know? What do you LIKE to do? What do you HAVE to do? What are you going to do next?

You are accountable for the answers to all of these questions. You direct your actions, and you determine how the actor (your body) will move through the TV show (your life). Whatever situation you find yourself in has been influenced by what you wanted for your life, the choices you made, and where you directed your attention and energy. *You will want to make friends with your director*. The director is in charge of casting and determines the quality of people you will surround yourself with. The director can request a new script or reassign the camera operator.

You can thank, yell at, or feel indifferent towards your "inner director" for your current state of affairs. Sure, you were born into a situation, the result of other people's decisions. You are the product of a million, billion random events from the past, in a world of billions of people trying to impose their will on their TV show. As a child, you were carried around, taken care of, schooled, somewhat shown the ways of the world, thrown into this or that group, and allowed to move about with limited autonomy. It was what it was.

Now, here you are, master of your universe, captain of your ship, seeker of truth and happiness...or not. You have been handed a blank page with the following heading at the top:

**“The Future: To Whom It May Concern”**

Now you get to fill up the empty space on the page. Actually, the page is not blank; penciled in are all of the stands you made in the past and the identities you assumed from childhood interpretations of what you experienced. (For example: "I'm this kind of person.", "I'm good at this, not good at that.") On the page is the script you have written as the scriptwriter...your future according to your past, colored with all the beliefs, preconceived notions, assumptions and habits you incorporated from other people and your experiences up to this point. Look at your page...where you are headed in the future has been penciled in. If it is not where you want to be, you will have to take a different approach.

"Whoa! Hold on one minute, can we go back to that pleasure cruise thing? Can I sit under a shade tree and just think of nothing for a while?"

"Sure, but that's what Rip Van Winkle said, so be forewarned."

"I know that story. The aimless, ambitionless Rip wanders in to the forest to get away from his belligerent wife, and falls asleep for 20 years under some spell. When he awakens, his life is behind him."

"Oh, that time thing. How much time do I have left?"

"You will never know."

"A sense of urgency?"

"It wouldn't hurt."

"And what about the ending?"

"I can't tell you."

"Can I live in a perfect fantasy?"

"It won’t help."

"So, I'm the main character; it's all about me?"

"Yep, at least that's what I tell everyone."

"And that pain and pleasure thing?”

"You'll figure it out."

"So how do I...?"

"It’s in the next chapters."

People love a good story. Did you notice the shift from being spoken to as the reader, to being in the audience, witnessing a dialogue? That is what we do. That's what happens to us as we experience our life. We start talking to ourselves, asking ourselves questions, trying to figure everything out. That is where the critic in us can begin to cause trouble. The “inner critic” is the voice in our head that judges and pre-judges all the feeling, seeing, hearing, smelling, tasting, and touching that we do, based on our current beliefs. While the critic describes our experiences with limiting names, labels, and rules, sometimes it is easy for us to forget that what the critic says is really just one opinion...not fact or truth. One of the most important skills you can learn is to completely silence the critic and decide for yourself whether you like the story of your life as it is unfolding.

# Chapter 3 - bringing awareness

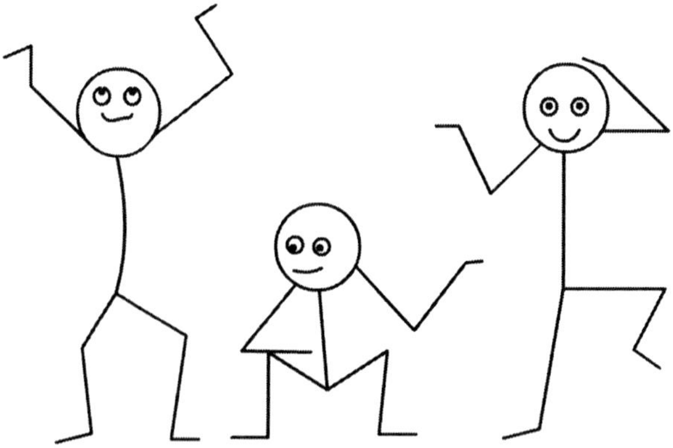

Now that you have begun the process of looking within (or at least thought about it!) let's focus those new self-investigation skills on a few specific areas. First, we will look at the idea of identifying the characteristics of your feelings, thoughts, reactions and actions in any given moment. We could call that "who you are being", but instead let's call that "how you are being" (there is an important distinction that we will examine in a little while).

Within this context, the description of "how you are being" at the time a situation is occurring can include:

- What you are thinking
- How you are feeling
- What you are saying/doing
- What you are telling yourself about your thoughts, feelings, words and actions

As you either witness or recall your thoughts, feelings, words, and actions, would you describe them, and you, as gentle, kind, confrontational, harsh, happy, frustrated, optimistic, depressed, content, dissatisfied, or resigned? Are you being Resistant? Convincing? Receptive? Defensive? Protective? Loving? Controlling? Engaging? Avoidant? Manipulative? Adaptable? Withholding? Open-hearted? Prevailing?

When you observe "how you are being", do you see yourself reacting to the past? Or are you maintaining your focus in the present and creating a healthy action instead of a reaction? Are you assuming a "role" to achieve some perceived purpose or are you able to express your real feelings about that moment?

Often we do not even want to identify or label how we are being, because we might not like what we find out about ourselves or don't want to examine why we are being that way. It is important that you approach this act of self-witness from an objective viewpoint, without judgment or "beating yourself up" for what you might see.

Even the most seemingly "negative" or "hurtful" way of being is, at some level, about helping us survive. Whether "how we are being" is about summoning our power or resisting a situation, our goal is to defend and protect the identity that we have created about ourselves. Whenever we are holding on to a part of our identity, living out the beliefs that we have taken on from the world around us, or looking to protect our perspective and point of view, how we are being is often simply a defense mechanism.

However painful and limiting they may be, defense mechanisms serve us until we decide we do not need them anymore. Deciding when that moment comes, and letting go of what no longer serves, is part of the process of becoming a "joyful being".

Earlier we made a distinction between "how we are being" and "who we are being". When we looked at "how we are being", we were describing some momentary aspect of our inner or outer experience. But when we describe "who we are being", it is all too easy to take on those descriptions as our long-term identity. When we ask "who we are being", the most common reply begins with the words "I am". I am angry...I am happy...I am frustrated...I am sad. The words "I am" are a statement about WHO YOU ARE, not just how you are feeling or behaving. When you say "I am sad", you are no longer saying that you are feeling sad in that moment. You are claiming being a sad person as part of your identity.

> **Example**: *You are at the grocery store with your child. You are in a hurry, rushing around to get what you need and get out. Your child sees his or her favorite type of colorful, sugary, cartoon-character-on-the-front, prize-in-the-box cereal and loudly and repeatedly pleads, begs, and demands that you buy it. The more frustrated and frazzled you feel, the louder and more persistent your child gets, maybe even to the point of a full-blown tantrum (yes, it happens to all us parents at one point or another...admit it, we even did it when we were kids). At that moment, you may snap and say something you*

*regret. Now, in that moment, you may very well think your child is beyond handling, and your child may very well be that difficult. But is your child that way all the time? Or is your child simply behaving like that in that moment? Is that your child's identity, or a description of five minutes of behavior?*

**Example:** *It is the middle of winter, cold and flu season. As much as you tried to avoid it, you have now picked up the bug that was being passed around the workplace...congested, coughing, head pounding, body aching...the whole thing. What do you say to yourself or to others about your current condition? Do you say "I have the flu?" or do you say "I am sick?" Maybe both? It is not something we think about often, but when we say "I have", there is an implication that right now it is in your possession but that might not always be the case. You may have $20 in your wallet right now, but did you always? And will you always? So you may "have" the flu right now or for the next few days, but most likely you will not have it for the rest of your life. But if you say "I am sick", you are saying "I am a sick person". Is it possible to be both a sick person and a "well" person at the same time? Are you claiming "sick person" as your identity?*

Through these examples it might seem like you are being asked to watch every thought you have and every word you speak. While a certain level of self-awareness is healthy and very beneficial on your journey, and you may even find yourself going overboard in the beginning as you learn these new awareness skills, the point is not about policing, editing, and censoring yourself in every moment. The point is simply about beginning to realize how much we humans create our experience of ourselves and our lives in each and every thought we have, word we speak, and action that we take. From that realization, you can begin to see just how much power, influence, and choice you have about the life you are living and the direction it is heading.

The problem with describing "who we are" and using "I am" statements is all too often we are doing so in a negative, limiting way, reinforcing beliefs about ourselves that we took on from others or decided for ourselves based on experiences in the past. Thinking or speaking one "I am sick" statement is not going to permanently change the course of your physical health forever. But how often do we tell ourselves "I am ugly", "I am fat", "I am unlovable", "I am lonely", "I am stupid", "I am broke/poor", "I am damaged/defective"? How many times each and every day do thoughts like that go through your head without you even noticing, because the tapes have been playing on repeat for the last 5, 10, 15, 20, 50 years of your life?

Just for a moment, try one of these "I am" statements on for size, observing your thoughts, feelings, and even body sensations as you think them to yourself or say them out loud to yourself:

- "I am lovable"
- "I am magnificent"
- "I am beautiful, inside and out"
- "I am intelligent and successful"

Did you believe what you thought/said? Or did some other voice pop in with "yeah, right, who are you kidding"? Did your body feel comforted and relaxed or did you get tense, maybe even nauseated, because the new message did not fit with what you already believe about yourself?

Through your cultivation of awareness you are able to identify both "how" and "who" you are being, and the awareness of your "being" provides you with new choices, alternatives, possibilities, and the opportunity for healthy actions. Bringing awareness to the constant stream of "I am" messages we tell ourselves about ourselves every day, in all their various forms, and to the power that "I am" statements have to transform our lives for the worse or the better, allows us to begin creating a new identity for ourselves...one that is based not on past messages from the world around us, but on who we authentically are and want to be.

# .Chapter 4 - staying in the present moment

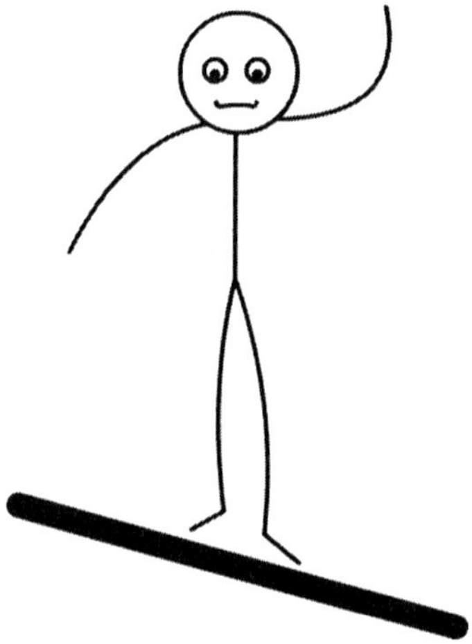

One of the easiest ways we can enjoy life is to take each moment as it comes. We are free to see each moment as a new and inviting opportunity. Keep it simple. Feel the sun on your face, breathe in the oxygen the trees give for free, walk on the ground that is always here for you to rest on. You are in a safe place and filled with a wealth of energy that surrounds you. You can draw from unlimited resources to be as you like. Every day is a chance to play, create, learn, love, and feel glad. Find the benefit in every situation. Remember, even in darkness you get to see the stars at night.

Most people say "who they are" in the present has everything to do with their past, including how they were raised, what school they went to, and how much money they had growing up. Most will be able to describe or label their history as being rich or poor, loved or unloved, etc. Amazingly, and contrary to any immediate logic, who you are in the present really has nothing to do with your past and everything to do with "the future you are looking into"! This statement seems peculiar at first, until you trace how and why you react in the present and where time in the past and future fit into your thoughts and reactions.

How did you become the person you are now? You would most likely say "from my life's events up to now". And with this you are describing the past. It seems obvious that the way you got to be the way you are is from the past. But what if I tell you that your past has nothing to do with your present? How can that be? Aren't we shaped by our experiences? How you view and project your future for yourself really controls your present. Yes, you can project your past onto your future, but what are you doing to yourself when you do?

Often it is not the past experience itself, but the painful emotions, stories, and beliefs that we continue to carry about the experience that we project into the future. It is not about forgetting the past; it is about putting down the burdens we continue to carry from the past. In upcoming chapters we will explore ways to release the emotional charges that you might still carry from past situations and interactions. By freeing yourself from those emotions, stories and beliefs, your past can become simply a collection of experiences you have had up to now, and your future can be powered by living in the present.

> **Example**: *It is 1:00 pm on a Friday, with 4 hours until you leave your job for the weekend. Looking at all the remaining work to be done, you get depressed thinking about how time will slow down until it is time to leave. Then you get a call from a friend who has an extra ticket to a Sunday concert. "Would you like to go?" For the rest of the day you think about the concert's sights and sounds, what you will wear, who you will see. Even though you are still at work, you are so excited! All day Saturday you do chores at home while thinking about the concert. Finally you get to the concert Sunday night and it is great! But while there, suddenly your thoughts shift to returning to work the next day, and you are back to the same low mood while you are still at the concert. It was not where you were or what you were doing that determined your mood, it was the thoughts you were thinking. Can you see now how your present is made up of the future you are projecting into, and not based on your past?*

Inner conversation or self-talk is continuous. This does not mean to suggest there is a necessity to suppress it. The goal is to gain mastery over the "noise" portion, such as the negative conversations you have with yourself, which direct you away from experiencing the present moment. The good news here is that most of the "noise", dialogues, self-talk, etc. you have are purely habit. You have been doing it for so long that you actually depend on it to avoid, justify, or excuse being responsible for the present moment.

If your mind is not in a state of peace you can be in the best situations and still not be happy. As you know now, happiness is really a state of mind! So, to break the habit of the mental "noise", you can practice letting go of the stories you are so busy telling yourself, turn off the "TV shows" in your head, and escape the "noise". At that moment you learn to enjoy the experience of living in the now.

As a condition of our existence we find ourselves in a constant state of need. We need air, food, water, warmth, money, and safety. We need love, acceptance, and achievement in our lives. We are subjected to external forces beyond our control, economic realities, physical limitations, and the demands of daily living. It seems we constantly want, desire, and wish for a never ending list of things. We love what we decided to love and we revel in anticipation of it. We want relief from anxiety, worry, fear, sadness, distress, boredom, disappointment, and frustration. We want to increase the pleasure, satisfaction, opportunities, choices, and well-being in our lives.

We may even want opposite things at the same time. We want to make money and we want free time, we want adventure and we want safety, and we want variety but we also want familiarity. Within these conflicts lies the paradox of our lives. We want and we want it now. We want instant gratification. However, "wanting" and "anticipating", no matter how fantastic the object of our desire may be, takes us out of the present moment and into the future that has not yet come. Ultimately all we ever have is now, and what we are creating now is like either planting a seed or not planting a seed. What seeds are you planting?

Our minds are programmed to deny, rationalize, and justify our actions and the consequences. We do not give up what we believe easily, or without effort, where we have a strong belief. We have the ability to rationalize just about anything, regardless of the overwhelming evidence to the contrary. We become scattered in our thoughts and make decisions that are not in our best interest. We can become unreliable, perform poorly at work, become manipulative in our relationships, and begin to blame everyone, including ourselves, harshly.

Sometimes we respond to what happens to us the way we think we should respond, as if it is the only way, and we have no choice. Difficulties happen to successful people, smart people, talented people, socially connected people, and people of all walks of life. No one is immune, and no one should expect to be immune. No one avoids frustration and disappointment in their life. But the effects can be minimized by our response.

Making our happiness conditional on things outside of our control or tied to things that have happened a long time ago is paralyzing. Being kind to ourselves, making time to calm the mind, and creating flexibility in our thoughts and bodies will help us instantly and in the long run.

It is incredibly cruel of us to think of ourselves in terms of negativity. We will see that thinking in terms of what we can't do, what we don't have, and what we don't want to happen is to some extent adversely contributing to our situation. By making friends with ourselves, seeing this type of behavior as abusive, and making an effort to change our self talk, we learn to accept the painful aspects of life that are beyond our control, and to take effective action to benefit ourselves and others.

By pausing, and taking a deep breath, we are reminded that the situation is just what's happening now. By mastering our breathing and calming response to distress we allow ourselves the freedom of choice. We can change what we do next instead of defaulting into habitual patterns that could harm us and limiting possibilities that don't serve us. We get stuck by avoiding and escaping, motivated by fear. With acceptance and the focusing of our attention we gain clarity of mind and the ability to respond appropriately to what has happened.

**Example**: *In grade school, while sitting in the classroom, your teacher asks for volunteers to answer a question, and you eagerly raise your hand. When called upon, your answer is wrong, and the entire class laughs at you. You tell yourself as a child "I will never make a fool of myself again". Now, as an adult, you avoid volunteering to speak up about anything. You* *avoid situations, places, people where you may have to answer a question or express an opinion. With this, you create your future and live in your adult present as if you were still in the grade school past.*

Allowing your past rejections, stories, and stands to sit out there in your future shapes your life in a way that does not allow you to be fair to yourself. You cheat your goals, needs, feelings, and thoughts, and may even stop yourself from fulfilling the possibilities you desire for your life. Do you notice how easy it is to set goals like I would like to do________ or be________? Many of us make statements like these every January 1st and call them "New Year's resolutions". But how many times do we actually make these dreams and goals happen? We know what to do, but we still cannot get things done. Sometimes our dreams do not come true because we have not yet cleared up the stories in our own minds concerning our past experiences.

Stop the re-telling of old stories and avoid seeking future stories to create. Without stories attached to your thinking, you are left with just the present moment. This act spontaneously connects you to your true inner self.

Worry or fear about the future means you are living in the future and not in the present. You worry because it somehow feels like you are "doing something" about the situation, but all you are really doing is moving yourself away from the place of calmness and clarity that allows you to see options and make the best decisions. That place can only be found when you are living in the present moment.

When your mind is in a state of worries, hopelessness, frustration, or any other mental discomfort you can bring it back into the peaceful state so important, on so many levels, for your own health and well-being. As you train your mind, you can be your own observer rather than a reactor. You can be in the frame of mind that brings positive results rather than being stuck in "reaction mode".

Your thoughts, actions and reactions reflect the Positive Mind, Negative Mind, and the Neutral Mind. The eternal optimist lives constantly in the Positive Mind until they are finally disappointed, and their hurt is profound. The pessimist, living in the Negative Mind, always expects the worst and usually gets it, with the best events passing by unnoticed.

Both the Positive and Negative minds usually come from reactive thinking. The Positive Mind stretches you beyond your perceived capabilities, and the Negative Mind protects you against the unseen dangers. But it is the Neutral Mind that allows you to take in life as it unfolds, absorbing and considering what you see and feel carefully and following-up with actions that you can truly claim as your own.

Neutral Minds find the most accurate solution for the situations around them. You can be a victim of your mind, falling prey to the fiction it creates, or you can have your mind be your best friend, providing options and understandings that are beneficial and accurate for the conditions at hand. The Neutral Mind can only be accessed when you are living in the present moment. Your goal is to achieve a Neutral Mind in which you are in a balanced state (even surrounded by chaos). You will simply be an observer with a non-judging mind. The cup won't be half full. The cup won't be half empty. It will just be a cup!

The technique for finding your way to a balanced, neutral mind and coming into the present moment is an interesting combination of a simultaneous "letting go" and a conscious act. Some call it centering, some simply call it calming down. The physical portion of this process is supported by the breathing and relaxation techniques provided in more detail in the upcoming chapters of this book. But, in short, through a purposeful combination of deep breathing, relaxing the body, becoming aware of the sensations and allowing a release of thoughts of the past and future, a gateway to the present opens up for decisions to be formed.

Through this process, you can move from a scattered, emotional, reaction state to a balanced, composed, action state. Through this process, you may receive an insight for resolution, a release of a "stuck issue", or the gift of a new perspective. The present moment becomes freed from the tedious cycles of "reacting to the reactions", of obsessing about the past, or fearing the future.

**Example**: *You are entering a train station, on your way to a very important meeting. You have just enough time to get to your appointment. Just as you are ready to step on to the train, the door closes in front of you. You look at the conductor like he closed the door on you on purpose, and you think or say "No!". Now you are in that stuck, resisting, reactive state of mind, thinking "why did this have to happen now" or "I can't believe this is happening to me". Anger has just risen and the mind gets stuck. Remember, stress is the tension that arises from the conflict between what we want to happen and what has happened. When you have a balanced, calm mind you have a solution-oriented mind and can consider options such as waiting for the next train or taking a cab or bus.*

In each aspect of awareness there is the physical component of settling in, or centering yourself, to let the thoughts come and go easily. You control your breathing; you allow your body to separate for just a moment from the activity of your thoughts. Then, once you have created that small, brief peace in your body, you allow your body to rejoin your thoughts and from a calmer place, witness "who" and "how" you are being.

Your first encounter with achieving a neutral mind through breathing and posture is usually after it is too late. You have already been caught in the anxiety and dramas of the moment, lost your composure, and have tried to recover to some functional state.

Your behavior is still all reaction. The next time you are confronted with a distress, you meet it more calmly, but eventually make a decision based on reaction. Finally, with additional experience, you come to a place where you can maintain calmness and a neutral mind. You become the observer of both yourself and the conditions around you. And then you act. You guide yourself, as a neutral observer of yourself, breathing and centering in that present moment. You guide rather than be guided.

When you are in the present moment and have a mind that is in balance you can see your options clearly and make decisions that benefit you. Be in balance and be ready for whatever life brings.

> **Example**: *We love the heroic stories of the Fireman, who, deep inside the burning building, clutches the baby under his protective jacket. He breathes from his emergency oxygen tank, and then alternates to breathe the air back into the baby's mouth. Fire sweeps by his body, and the lumber crashes around him. He emerges outside, baby saved, crowds applauding, a hero. This is the stuff movies are made of, but we know it has occurred in real life. Reports from these remarkable persons show that during such a crisis, time seems to slow down, a sense of calm occurs, and each action occupies its own moment. The incident becomes just a series of moments performed with effortless clarity.*

Taking action with calmness and clarity, based on a series of present moments...does that sound like what we have discussed so far? When we look at it in such dramatic terms, it seems that we can achieve this state because our lives depend on it. But when we place it in the realm of everyday life, it seems there is not as much motivation as being trapped in a burning building.

But guess what? Your life literally does depend on living in the present moment. You can become your own hero, creating calm, emotional postures; seeing with clarity and perspective; and taking action instead of reacting. Learn to love the present moment and be your own hero!

# Chapter 5 - calming the mind

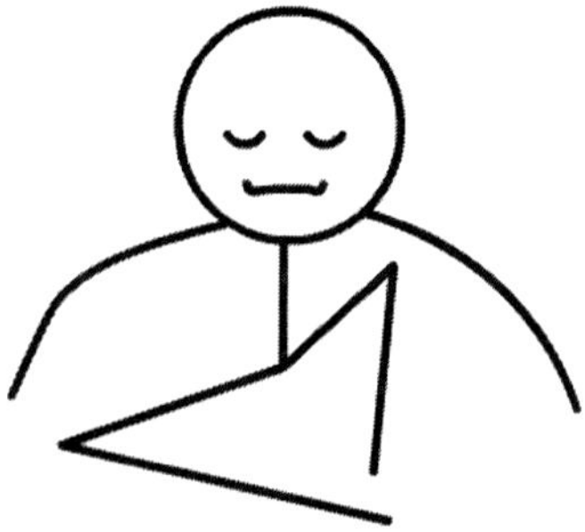

When you are in an emotional state, you cannot think straight or sometimes at all. Love is blind. Hate is crippling. Fear freezes us in time. When you are controlled by your emotions, your ability to gather evidence and make the most beneficial choice is impaired. It is the same when you are stressed out. Stress can come from having your car break down on the highway, having two appointments in different places at the same time, your boss giving you more work to complete by Monday, or your partner complaining about you not having enough free time to give. Stress is a condition of anxiety caused by an inability, or perceived inability, to cope with a situation. It does not even have to be true, only thought or assumed to be so. Stress is the tension created by the difference between what is happening and what you want to happen.

Stress and pressure are not only terms to express your emotional feelings, these things are actually happening in your body. If you feel trapped in a traffic jam, in a relationship, or in a job, you feel an inability to successfully negotiate a change for the better in your life. Your heart works harder, your blood vessels become constricted, your body temperature rises, and you breathe more rapidly but get less oxygen with each shallow breath. By calming the mind, you are creating a peaceful space within yourself so you can see how you are being.

When you are in a stressed state, it is important to modify negative self-talk into comforting and encouraging statements. However, because of the physical stress reaction in your body, this is not always easy to do. Instead, you can start by controlling your breathing. It is not as simple as "just breathe". You are already breathing. It is an awareness of *how* you are breathing. You could be breathing too much and hyperventilating, or you may have held your breath in a gasp without realizing it.

Bringing attention to your breathing shows you are in control, and is a very powerful tool for generating a real state of calm. Using breathing in this way is at first purposeful, but can also become a natural part of your response mechanisms in a whole range of emotional scenarios. First, breathing must be developed as a skill by taking small amounts of time in each day to practice specific breathing techniques. Even after these techniques become part of your body's natural rhythm, taking time to practice conscious breathing exercises stimulates your body's systems, invigorates your concentration, and provides a reservoir of calmness for the remainder of the day!

The “three-part-breath” (diaphragmatic breathing) exercise below is a good place to start. By breathing the complete breath it utilizes the full capacity of the lungs. You will exchange more carbon dioxide for oxygen, and invigorate all the systems of the body. It is more than our lungs that breathe, every cell in our body needs oxygen to survive.

As you incorporate breath awareness into your life you will begin to recognize that often the restless, nervous sensations you feel in your body are actually the result of your thoughts and emotions. The physical desire to smoke a cigarette after eating a meal or the wound-up-ready-to-explode feeling in your body that leads you to pace around the room all really begin in your mind. When you observe your physical behavior you will notice that no act or gesture occurs independently of the mind. The mind always moves first then the body follows.

Just being conscious of breathing contributes to gaining a peaceful mind and undisturbed state. When the breath begins to move evenly, effortlessly and quietly through the nostrils without hesitation, the mind begins to settle in to a quieter and more serene place. This stillness sets the mind free to differentiate between what is ego and what is inspiration, approaching a deeper concentration some would term as a meditation.

## *Diaphragmatic Breathing*

Regulated breath is always ruled by non-injury. Never take breathing beyond your comfort. Inhale or exhale as much air as possible within your capacity. With practice your capacity will increase, but this is not to be considered a contest to see how fast your body can adapt. Breath is the science of restoring the body's natural rhythms by learning not to breathe with only the upper chest; but rather by purposefully using the diaphragm. Be attentive to creating gentle, full, steady diaphragmatic breath. A complete and steady diaphragmatic breath is made up of three distinct phases involving the abdominal (belly), thoracic (mid-lung) and clavicle (upper-lung) regions. Diaphragmatic breathing is natural to a newborn baby. It's just automatic to them.

### ***EXERCISE:***

As you start your breathing exercise, when a thought comes simply recognize it as a thought, let it go, and bring your attention back to the breath. As you practice you will feel many thoughts and sensations come up, like "what was I doing?", "I'm hungry!", "what is so and so doing?", etc. Many thoughts will arise, but just bring yourself back to the present moment so you can do this exercise. As you learn to master your thoughts, you will be capable of mastering your reactions to frustrating, painful or uncomfortable situations.

Allow your body to automatically release the tension of what you want to happen and what is happening. This gives you the ability to have a mind that can produce a better outcome for you and your life, creating more health and well-being for yourself.

Let's begin your first breath exercise:

1. Take a seat, or you can stand where ever you are.

2. Make sure your spine is straight. Roll your shoulders back and down.

3. For diaphragmatic breathing, feel a "balloon" positioned just behind your belly button. When you inhale, the balloon fills your belly and gently moves outward. When you exhale, your balloon goes down gently.

4. Place your hands on your belly, inhale, and feel the palms of your hands lift up as your belly expands.

5. Exhale, feeling your hands lower again as you slowly contract (tighten) the abdominal muscles and squeeze out all of the residual air.

6. Shift your hands to the sides of your ribcage and repeat the inhale/exhale process, for your mid-lung section. Feel your ribcage expand as you inhale, and release all the residual air as you exhale.

7. Place your hands on your collarbone and again repeat the inhale/exhale process for the upper-lung section, feeling your collarbone, clavicle and first 3 ribs lift as you inhale and releasing all the residual air as you exhale.

8. Let your hands fall down to your side or rest on your legs, and inhale through the nose with the mouth closed if possible. Fill the lower lungs, then the mid-lung section, then the upper-lung section.

9. Slowly exhale as you contract the abdominal muscles and release all the residual air.

You can practice three-part-breath as an exercise in the morning, evening, or any time. Let your thoughts go and focus on the breathing only. Take 3 breaths, emphasizing each area of the lungs. Build up to 5 minutes for the total routine. Then, take deep breathes that start in the abdominal area, continuing to draw in air. Breathe out as if you have just been relieved of a burden.

This is how you can “de-stress” in any situation. You can find a place to retreat to in a situation or crisis, breathe, and recapture your sense of calm. When you are waiting in line, in traffic, or any time that frustration builds, take that one deep breath and continue as needed. This is how you center yourself and calm yourself down. This way of breathing brings more oxygen to your brain, bloodstream, and cells.

The remarkable thing is that if you include three-part-breath exercises into your daily routine, and you are later confronted with a crisis that doesn’t allow the time or place for the exercise, you can simply bring your attention to your breath, and the process of calm and centering will begin for you.

Calming the mind can be as simple as reminding yourself who is boss. You are the boss of your thinking, breathing, and body. Allowing your thoughts to run away with you is a choice you make. Being drawn into drama or chaos by others who may be manipulating you is a choice you make. Keep your power and your peace, don't give it away.

***Breathing is one of the most elemental parts of living.***
***It is the tool that maintains or recaptures***
***your power, life force, focus, balance, and direction.***

# Chapter 6 - letting go

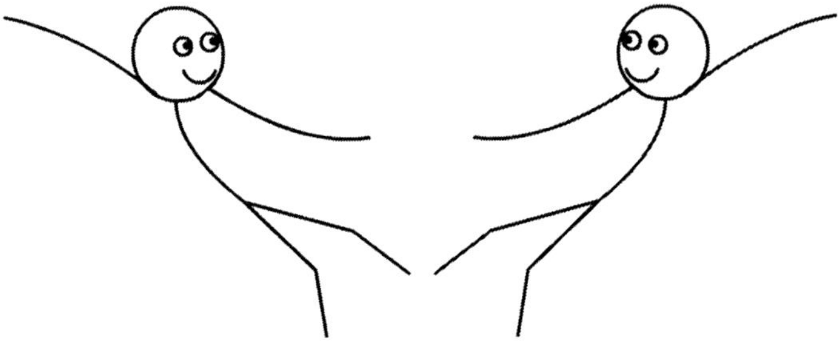

As you begin to gain the ability to calm your mind, explore your own thinking, and become a “self-witness” to your life, you also begin to notice that you also have the ability to make choices. Although you may typically think of choices in terms of the various things you can do, you might also consider the things you do not want to do. Ridding yourself of unwanted thoughts, or ways of thinking, is still a conscious act. Here we will call it “letting go”.

“Letting go” refers to letting go of the past. Not in the sense of forgetting, but in the sense of letting go of the pain and disappointment. It can also be called “releasing”, but in many ways it could also be called “surrendering”. Surrendering seems to connote letting something have the power over you, not take the power back. So how can this be “letting go”? And why can’t you “not do” something the old fashioned way, by just stubbornly refusing, or, even more classically, just pretending the issue or thought does not exist until it hopefully disappears? The answer is in the "why" you would let go in the first place…to eliminate tension, both emotionally and physically. Letting go happens on the emotional level, with the elimination of painful, hurtful feelings, and on the physical level, in the cells, muscles, spine, digestive system, and all other areas of the body. Our classic responses to frustrating and painful situations cause even more tension, so in using your classic responses you just replace one useless waste of energy with another.

So let's continue to look at why you would want to let go, to help you better understand the "how" of letting go. Often the rethinking of personal histories over and over again is referred to as "playing tapes in your head". I guess in modern terms you have to say playing CD's or DVD's in your head! Since this doesn't seem to have the same usefulness as the vision of playing, rewinding, playing, rewinding a tape recording, let's continue to envision the tape recorder. In this context, letting go means releasing the emotional charge of past experiences and not reliving them over and over again.

Letting go does not just apply to obsessive thoughts. It also applies to worrying if you have done something correctly in the past, lingering resentment for perceived harm done to you, re-living a sad or traumatic event, or fear about the future. The process of letting go can only occur in the present moment, when you bring awareness to a specific situation. Whether you are talking about past, future, or present events, it is in the present where you experience either the benefits of letting go or the damage of not letting go.

It is important to understand that NOT letting go also has an emotional pay-off. If you play the role of "victim", you may get sympathy and attention in a manipulative way. However, the benefits of this approach are far outweighed by the harmful long-term effects of holding yourself back and keeping yourself in pain. The decision of whether, and when, to let go is completely up to you.

Letting go of a situation does not mean that what a person did to you or what you did to someone else was ok. It does not mean that you have to stay in an unhealthy, painful situation. Letting go, or forgiveness, in this case, is the willingness to release the stored, toxic anger, blame and resentment and return to your natural state of health and well-being.

Why should you let go of certain thoughts or ways of thinking?

1. Distraction – you are not where you should be, in the present. Your mind is bouncing back and forth re-reading old scripts, re-writing new scripts, trying to get the story to come out in a way that will justify, satisfy, vindicate, or even condemn.

2. Tension – there is a contradiction and friction between what you feel inside about an issue and what you consciously perceive; or there is a contradiction between

what others around you express as their feelings and how you perceive the same event or issue.

3. Energy – You don't realize how the repeating cycle of these types of thoughts wear you down. Physically, mentally, emotionally you become fatigued, and your ability to resist adding even more useless thoughts and re-considerations continues, until most of your available energy is consumed "playing tapes".

When we talk about letting go, we do not mean forgetting an event ever happened or had no impact on our life. There is nothing wrong with reflecting back to good memories or using lessons learned from painful situations to shape our lives in positive ways. However, letting go of the emotional charges that come when we think about a situation frees us to more clearly see the situation, including any benefits and lessons we were given.

Letting go of the emotional charges means letting go of the power the event has over us. Even holding on to emotions connected to positive experiences can limit us. Have you ever had such a fun time that you thought "Wow, this was the best time ever! My life will never be this good again!"? When we have thoughts like that about an experience, we are basically telling ourselves life is all "downhill" from here, and then we seek out ways to re-create those experiences to get back to that great feeling, instead of being open to the next great experience.

When we attach to a specific experience, whether it be the "best ever" or "worst ever" we give that experience power over our peace of mind and ability to stay in the present moment. When we "let go" of those emotional charges, we are able to think about our experiences in more beneficial ways, such as:

1. Careful, slow considerations and thoughts: Whether you call it contemplation, introspection, or meditation, it is the process of getting to know your true, inner self and it involves the calm, deliberate consideration of past or future events for the purpose of determining an action or coming to a conclusion.

2. Remembering: The simple process of bringing forward as accurately as possible details, information, or events so that they can be organized for some purpose.

3. Communication: Your interaction with others and the back and forth communications that require considering alternate perspectives, clarifications, and conclusions.

It would be easy to conclude that it is our thoughts and thinking patterns that we need to let go of. However, it is really about letting go of those emotional charges and limiting beliefs about ourselves and our lives. Obsessively thinking about something is our mind's way of attempting to find an answer to the question of "how to stop feeling so horrible". When we let go, we will no longer feel "horrible" and the obsessive thinking is no longer needed.

If we simply tell ourselves to stop thinking about something, but still feel the pain, we are actually creating even more pain for ourselves by taking away our coping skills and maybe even beating ourselves up for our inability to "stop thinking about" something. Then, with that added pain, the vicious cycle continues and escalates.

How do you tell the difference between non-useful obsessive thoughts and thinking patterns and those functional "re-thoughts" that are required to make useful and/or beneficial decisions? If you take note of what occurs in useful and non-useful thoughts, the useful, whether it concerns the past, future or present, has an action being created in the present. The non-useful thoughts are fairly easily identified as just a series of reactions upon reactions that never provide a conclusion…only a return to the same rehashing of a thought, event, or literally the retelling of some story out of sheer habit.

Granted, habits can certainly work to your advantage; however, habits can also inhibit your ability to navigate the present or live into a useful future. By their very nature, habits are patterns of thinking or behavior that have been repeated so many times in the past that they are carried out almost unconsciously or involuntarily. When we are acting out of habit, we are no longer living with awareness and making choices in the present moment.

A good way to track the creation of habits is to look at why you had the thought or took the action in the first place. When did the habit begin? When the thought or action first occurred, why did you do it, and what benefit did you receive from doing it? In other words, why did you decide to do it again? Was it comfortable? Did you feel safe and secure? Was it fun? Was it the most convenient option? You made the decision the first time, perhaps "in the present moment" and perhaps not, but when you decided to repeat the thought or action, you made that decision based on the pay-off you received in the past. Then, when you received the same pay-off/benefit the second time, you did it again, and so on. From there, a habit was formed.

Now that you have looked at the types of things you want to let go of, let's begin letting go. First, become a "self-witness" to your actions. Make a conscious effort to see how you spend your time, your words, and your efforts. "How" and "who" are you being? Sad? Not enough? Devastated? Confused? Then, begin to note where you "spin your wheels" trying to accomplish a task, break a habit, or communicate a point to someone.

Pick out just one of these "stuck places" as an item to work on. For now, do not give any consideration to the thoughts invested in this. Make sure it is an area of life that is important to you. Categories could include family, relationships, finances, sex, and retirement. Look at that area of your life and ask yourself what qualities would make the difference in that area. Answers may include peace, joy, love, and communication.

Find a quiet place to be still. Begin to breathe in an even, yet full, inhalation and exhalation rhythm. Become aware of the various sounds, smells, and objects in your physical surrounding. One by one put them in the background, and concentrate on your breathing. Now bring up the single "stuck item" you have chosen for this exercise. As you begin to consider this "old friend", become your own witness to the recurring pattern of the story.

Often your story originates in childhood experiences. When you are a child, you think the world revolves around you. You don't see your parents as human beings with their own stories or perceptions. You see them for their roles in your life, as authority figures and as providers for your physical and emotional needs. Realize that this story is an old story, re-written, re-read, retold, in your thoughts over and over. When we think about how the future will be (either as a negative experience or a positive one) we are really repeating an old story and changing the setting to place it in a future context. It is not a future that will necessarily happen. It is an old story you have used to mask and limit the real possibilities in your life...the real future.

**Example**: *A young child who is not old enough to know the danger reaches to touch a hot stove. His mother grabs his hand just in time so he does not get burned. As the mother grabs the boy's hand she says "NO!" because she does not want her son to get burned. The child sees that his mother is upset, but does not realize that she is coming from her own*

> *perception of not wanting her child to get burned. The child runs it through his own little mind and his perceptions. The child's thought might be "mom's mad at me, she does not like me". This idea might then linger and influence how the child interprets his mother's words and actions in the future.*

Understand that nothing will change about a situation until you consciously decide to make a change. Nothing happens automatically while we sit by and wait, our action is required. Even in situations where you feel like a helpless victim, taking one small step or changing one thought to break the pattern initiates the process.

Now, it's time to play an imagination game. Imagine that "stuck item" as something you can hold (however big and heavy it might be). See yourself pick it up. Then see yourself turn around, put the item down, and turn back around again so the item is now where it belongs...behind you, in the past. See and feel that "stuck item" sitting there behind you, no longer being carried in your arms or sitting out there in the future in front of you.

Bring your awareness back to your breathing and your immediate surroundings. When you have put down and let go of your "stuck item", notice how that process feels to you. In the next chapters we will look at the process for releasing the emotional charges around the "stuck item" you are working with, but for now just be aware of any reactions and emotions you felt when you "saw" yourself putting the specific situation behind you.

When you give yourself permission to begin “letting go”, even the thought of doing so or symbolically beginning the process through this imagination game may bring up emotional reactions, including both fear (resistance) and relief. You may feel anger. You may spontaneously laugh. Tears may come. You may feel like the weight of the world was just lifted from your shoulders or you may feel completely lost and alone without this “old friend” there to keep you company. There is no “correct” or “incorrect” reaction, just notice what comes.

The goal is to have an awareness of the present and the possibilities in a real future take the place of that past story. If you were not willing to put the “stuck item” behind you when you first attempted to do so, that is ok. When you feel ready, try again, and see what happens. Even in our resistance, there is information. If we are not ready to let go of something it means that continuing to carry that “something” has a benefit for us in some way, and only when we understand that benefit can we truly decide to let go once and for all. Remember, including conscious breathing as you work through this exercise helps you center and calms you enough to do the exercise.

It’s important to note that in this exercise, no one, including yourself, needs to be assigned blame. No issue needs to be feared. No solution or conclusion about a “stuck item” needs to be made.

You are shifting away from the “blame, judgment and fear game” in your process of letting go. You are seeing that the distractions, tension, and depleted energy of your old stories have nothing to do with the people or situations involved. Allowing something in the past to hijack your present and future is the cause. You gave it permission. The good news is you can also give it permission to go back to where it belongs...in the past. There, it is in the appropriate place to become an event you can learn from, regret, and even mourn.

The best news of all is that once you put that story where it belongs, and only when you put that story where it belongs, you perform your most powerful act yet in letting go. You can forgive. Forgiveness is not about forgetting or letting someone "off the hook" for their words or actions in the past. Forgiveness means having the willingness to release the toxic energy of old stored anger, blame and resentment in your mind and body and to return to your natural state. Forgiveness is not done for the other person or situation, forgiveness is a gift you give yourself. When you forgive that other person or situation, it no longer has power over you.

Allow peace to enter you through the process of forgiveness. You can forgive others, those alive and departed. You can forgive misjudgments. And most of all you can forgive yourself, knowing you did the best you could in that situation with the information that was given to you at that time. You begin to shift, move forward, and see the real possibilities in your life. Nothing is ever lost by letting go. Everything is gained.

# Chapter 7 – when buttons are pushed

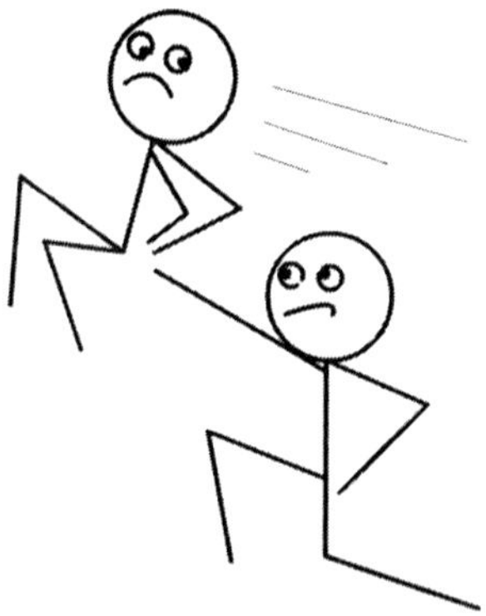

It's a great day. The sun is shining. You are having a "good hair day" or looking cute in the new shirt you recently bought at a great sale price. You just finished that big project at work and got praised for the fabulous job you did. You are having dinner later with some good friends that you have not seen for a while, and you know you will have a great time together. For a moment, all is well in your world. And then it happens.

It could be your parent, your brother or sister, your friend, your boyfriend/husband or girlfriend/wife, your co-worker or boss, or a stranger on the street. Whatever the case, someone somewhere says or does something, and in a split second all that warm, fuzzy, calm, centered, "life is great" feeling goes out the window and you are suddenly angry, sad, frustrated, vengeful, hostile, grumpy, judgmental, blaming, feeling victimized, and thinking thoughts like "life stinks!" and "why does something always happen to ruin my good mood?". Guess what! Your buttons just got pushed!

In previous chapters you have learned that self-exploration and self-awareness are tools you can use on your journey to becoming a "joyful being". You have also learned how powerful your thoughts and beliefs are in terms of how you see yourself and your life. You may have started to observe yourself in various situations, begun practicing conscious breathing to help calm and center yourself in moments of upset, and even experimented with the idea of putting past events behind you. Yet, once again, there is a moment where something happens and you are back in a reactive state.

When a "button" gets pushed, we think we are reacting or responding to the "something" that is happening in that moment. But, if you take a couple deep breaths and step back into observer mode, you will often see that the intensity of your reaction seems extreme for the situation itself. This observation is not about passing judgment on yourself or telling yourself you are "over-reacting", but about opening the door to ask the question "What is really going on here? What am I *really* reacting to?".

Remember all those beliefs, stories, and painful situations from the past that we have been looking at? You know, the ones with emotional charges that we carry with us into the present and project into the future? THOSE are our buttons! We carry our beliefs, stories and painful situations from the past with us as if they are both our identity and our protection. When something happens in the present that reminds us a little too much of the pain of the past, comes a little too close to threatening our beliefs, or validates and reinforces the negative things we already tell ourselves about ourselves every day, we react. We may not even consciously know what we are reacting to. The beliefs, stories, and painful situations might not even be in our conscious awareness. In fact, we might not even remember that the past experience ever happened. But it is there, and in that moment of reaction, it is running the show.

When you were young, you absorbed the world view demonstrated to you by your parents and others around you. At first it was "their" world, but more and more it became "your world", until that world outside yourself became indistinguishable from who you were inside. You formed your identity based on what had been explained to you as good or bad, as pretty or ugly, and as lovable or unlovable. You consciously or unconsciously claimed ownership of all the things you had been taught and came to believe in. Once you claimed it, you then decided to defend and protect it!

You built arguments in defense of your life story, as you would build a protective wall around your home. The trouble with walls is the higher and thicker you build them, the harder it is to see beyond them. Your parents and others told you stories, you believed them and allowed the stories to define you. You took ownership of the stories as part of who you were and then you needed to protect the stories from any opposition. Whew! That's a lot of work. No wonder we are all so tired all the time!

As you start to realize that your reactions are really just defenses to your buttons being pushed and begin to explore the hidden beliefs, stories and pain that are prompting the reactions, you can begin taking that wall down, brick by brick, at whatever pace feels comfortable and safe for you. It all begins with observation and awareness.

Who has been wronged or who is in the right during these "button-pushing" moments are not as important as being conscious of your own internal role and how little the people around you really have to do with your reactions. Your buttons being pushed can leave you tired, confused, frustrated and angry. However, you can learn to shift your perspective.

Have you ever said "You made me sad" or "that shopkeeper's attitude made me furious"? Does someone else's behavior actually make you feel a certain way? If so, then you believe that someone else has complete control over you...your feelings, your thoughts, your behavior, and your peace of mind. Otherwise, how else could they "make you" anything? When you say someone's words, actions, or mere existence "makes you" feel or respond in a certain way, you are giving your power away to that other person or situation. When you give your power away, you become reactive instead of proactive, and you have reactions instead of taking action that is in your best interest in a conscious, clear-headed way.

In Chapter 3 – Bringing Awareness, you looked at the idea of how powerful your thoughts and words can be. We discussed how repeatedly using the words "I am" to describe a temporary experience (I am sad, I am hungry, I am sick) shifts the description of that experience to a limiting description of your identity. The same thing can be said about the idea of someone or something else "making you" feel or do anything. Whenever you think or say those words, you are reinforcing to yourself that the world, and other people, have control of your life and your peace of mind. What starts out as a harmless expression can, when used often enough, impact how you see yourself and your experiences in life.

Have you ever told someone you love that they "make you happy"? Even in those positive experiences and moments, you are surrendering your power and peace of mind to someone else. If having someone specific in your life is what "makes you" happy, what happens to your state of happiness for the rest of your life if that person is no longer there? When you believe your happiness (or any other desired quality of life) is dependent on someone else's presence or behavior, you react to any perceived threat to your relationship with that person as a threat to your happiness. Stress, sadness, a sense of helplessness, jealousy, control issues, abuse issues, fighting to get someone to be who you want them to be (instead of accepting who they are), and much more can result when you believe someone else has the power to control your quality of life.

As a child, did your parent or some other significant adult in your life ever say you "made them happy" or "made them mad"? Didn't you then decide to base at least some of your behavior and choices for your life on their anticipated response? Whether it was following the rules for being part of your family or rebelling against them, you were given the message that you had power over someone else's life. You possibly even altered how you lived your life (giving up your personal power in the process) while that person never saw the impact of those words on themselves or on you, never claimed their own personal power, and never took responsibility for their own thoughts, words and actions.

Another way we give our personal power up to outside circumstances and stay in a "buttons-pushed" reactive state is by arguing with reality. How many times each day do you think or say something like "I should exercise more", "He/she should treat me with respect", "I shouldn't think or feel that way about something", or "People shouldn't treat each other cruelly"? When you use the words "should" and "should not", or their cousins "must", "must not", "supposed to", "not supposed to", "have to", and other variations on arbitrary rules, you are basically saying that reality is not acceptable. You get upset and believe you will not be "ok" again until those circumstances change.

When you resist and argue with reality, you spend your mental, emotional and sometimes physical energy trying to change reality and what has already taken place. If your peace of mind is dependent on a person, place or thing changing or some past event being "undone" you have given your personal power away to that person, place, thing, or past event. Only when you accept what has happened as "reality" do you free yourself to clearly assess your options and take action to create more favorable outcomes in the future. Accepting reality does not mean you have to like what happened. But until you say "yes, it happened, now what am I going to do about it from here?", you will never be able to move past "it".

It is important to understand that every person has buttons that get pushed at one point or another. We all have pain from the past, we all have beliefs that we have taken on from others, and we all have stories about who we are and how the world works. When we begin taking responsibility for the way our life is unfolding by practicing self-awareness, doing the work to shift the limiting thoughts, beliefs and stories, and releasing the emotional pain we carry from past events, it is very easy, and very common, to start judging ourselves even more for "how messed up we are" or "how slowly we are making the changes". We might even look at someone else's life and compare "stories", deciding who had the worst experience, has more "stuff" to work through, or who had it easier.

Everyone has their own individual life to live, including their own individual perceptions and interpretations of events in their lives. Everyone goes at their own pace, in whatever way is comfortable, safe, and best for them. It may sound cliché and at the same time hard to believe, but at each moment we really are "where we are supposed to be". It is not about comparison and competition...that is just one more story that we tell ourselves about ourselves and just one more way we abuse ourselves. And while you may now be thinking "See, I messed up again! When will I ever learn?", having our buttons pushed is really an opportunity for transformation.

If we didn't have the button pushed, we might not even know it was there, still having control over our experiences in life. Take that breath, go into observation mode, and bring awareness to what is really happening and what you are really reacting to. Laugh with yourself, say "Oops! I did it again!", and take that opportunity for self-awareness as an opportunity for a fresh start in life...even if it happens 20 times a day.

In the first century, Epictetus, an ancient Greek philosopher, wrote: "Men are disturbed not by things, but by the views which they take of them." Much of our stress, emotional pain and reactivity come from our thoughts about a situation and not the situation itself. On one level, realizing that it all comes down to "you" can be frustrating and overwhelming. You may even choose to hold on to your "victim" identity a while longer so as to not have to start doing the work for yourself.

However, on another, deeper level, realizing that you, and only you, have the power to change your life for the better can be completely empowering and liberating. Simply by accepting the current situation as "reality", releasing the pain of the past, deciding what beliefs are truly yours and letting go of the rest, and rewriting your stories, you can change your perceptions of life...which will change your thoughts about past, current and future events... which will set you free.

One way to begin shifting from a reactive state to an empowered state involves all those arbitrary rules we looked at earlier...all the "should", "supposed to", "must", and "have to" statements and the "not" statements that go with them. We know now that in order to create a different situation in the future, we first need to accept that what is, *is*. What happened, *happened*. It may change in the future, or it may not. The person who just "dumped" you or the boss who just fired you may very well change their mind and take you back. The person who just insulted or disrespected you may very well apologize. But if you are waiting for that to happen in order to feel safe, secure and happy in the world again, you may be in for a hard time ahead.

Acceptance of a situation does not require or equal approval of a situation. We may not like someone's behavior, but we can avoid the emotional stress of resisting reality by accepting it as "what is" without approving of it. We may not like our current reality, but by changing our rules about how life "should" be to a preference for how we would *like* life to be, we take back our power.

When we say "should" or "should not", we get reactive when the world does not follow our rules of conduct. When we say "I would prefer if", we are stating a personal opinion. Then, when the world does not comply, we may be disappointed but we are not stuck in the mode of resisting what "is". When, for the moment, the situation cannot be changed to something that better suits you, then climb that emotional hill as described in the next chapter. Accept the reality of the situation, breathe, relax, feel the feelings of sadness, anger, disappointment or frustration and their accompanying physical sensations run through your body, and then let them go. Once you have moved from a reactive state to a calm, centered state, you can then begin to look at your options and make the best decision on how to proceed.

> **Example**: *When experiencing a loss, one person's inner dialogue or "self-talk" might be: "It's unfortunate this happened. I have no reason why it occurred. It's sad that this happened, but it is not awful and I can continue to function". Another person might use the following "self-talk": "This absolutely should not have happened and it is horrific that it did. These circumstances are intolerable and I cannot continue to function." The first person's response is apt to lead to sadness, while the second person may well be on his way to depression.*

When your buttons get pushed, another way to shift from a reactive state to an empowered state is by identifying then challenging the negative thoughts and self-talk that caused the painful feelings about a situation.

Examine the actions that you took. Once you have identified the buttons that were pushed, including the thoughts and feelings you had about all aspects of the situation, you can then challenge your beliefs, thoughts, and self-talk to see if they are "true". From there, you can identify alternative beliefs, thoughts and behaviors that are more positive and self-nurturing.

After someone or something pushes your buttons, ask yourself the following questions about the event:

**What is the specific situation or event**?

**What are your feelings about the event?** Are you depressed and/or angry? How old do you feel? Does the situation itself, or the way you feel about the situation, remind you of similar experiences in the past? These questions may help you identify that your reactions to the current event are really related to unresolved feelings and beliefs that originated from past experiences. Identifying the age helps you to see that your emotional response may be connected to your past history. As you repeat this exercise, you may see patterns, especially in relation to the age you feel when certain buttons get pushed. You can then work on healing those past wounds and not continue to blame people and events in the present for your feelings and behaviors.

**How are you behaving as a result of the event?** You may cry, overeat and do self-destructive things or you may lash out in rage and do or say things you may regret.

**What are your beliefs about the event - your self-talk (the stories you created based on your perception of the event)?** "I feel so abandoned, rejected, stupid, worthless, I have no control over my life, no one loves me, no one values me, etc." (resulting in depression) or "This is awful, everything happens to me, the world is so unfair" (resulting in hostility)

**In what ways can you dispute the stories you created about the event?** Question your beliefs and self-talk about the situation. This is where you take your power back by recognizing the other person is not responsible for what you are feeling. Look at the stands you made when you felt the same way as a child, teenager, or younger adult. When you take full responsibility for what you are feeling, you can walk away from the lessons that were learned without continuing to repeat and be limited by the story; i.e. "Where's the evidence that I'm a worthless person?"

**What are your new, more empowered feelings about the event?** Recognize, own, and re-write the script of the story that was created by your previous perceptions (not enough, etc.) i.e. "I have so much to offer and when I choose to love and value myself I will experience that in the world as well" or "The world is full of injustices. It is what it is. I can accept what I can't change."

**What are your new/future behaviors as a result of the event?**

1. You may recognize the need to take a look at the stories that you created based on your belief systems.
2. You may begin to recognize that no one but you can make you happy and begin to set healthier boundaries in relationships.

Taking the time to really look at the button that was pushed and question the real reason for your reactions is the first step in healing the pain. If you only address the current situation, the button remains. When you really look at, re-script, and release the pain of the original event, there is no more emotional charge and the "button" will no longer be there to be pushed.

Look at where you feel victimized. Where did you reject yourself? Look at things in context instead of going through life and reacting to the situations out of habit or conditioning or as your buttons are being continuously pushed. Look at "the story of me" without carrying the identity of it anymore.

Look at the situation as simply something that happened in the past, where you are no longer in a reactive relationship to those events or seeking a remedy from the relationship within the story of the past (ex: what he/she did to me). You no longer need it as a definition of who you are. You can look at the future with a different perspective of "who you are being" as you create your future without the anxiety, fear and rejection. Not to say you will not have challenges in the future (we all do!), but that you will be freed to handle the challenges in the present moment instead of as a reaction based in and on past experiences. You will have the strength and power to deal with the situation in the moment with healthy actions, not just reactions. As any situation arises that needs to be dealt with you can handle it in a calm, collective way rather than a reactive way. When you take the time to heal and release the past, you give yourself the gift of freedom.

# Chapter 8 - climbing the emotional hill

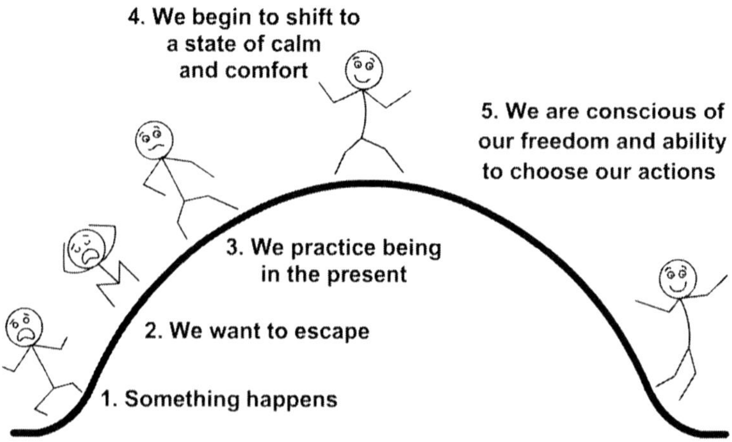


When life comes at you quickly and unexpectedly, what do you do? What do you do when you feel overwhelmed emotionally? The events of daily life can range anywhere from easy to overwhelmingly difficult. The resulting feelings and physical reactions, depending on your perception of the severity of the events, can leave you stuck at the bottom of an emotional hill without the means to climb to a comfortable place on the other side. You can either judge how "bad" or how "not so bad" a particular incident is and get lost in whether you need to panic, hide, or ignore it…or you can just go ahead and climb the emotional hill.

Let's look at the different stages of this "hill climbing process in a little more detail:

1. Something happens:
   You are confronted with an incident, with no immediate means of resolution. It takes on a sense of seriousness, worry, weight, or threat. It is, in any case, enough to cause you distraction or distress.

2. We want to escape:
   Without a ready and acceptable solution, what do you do? How do you try to escape the situation? Do you collapse, hide, shut your eyes tight, curl up in a corner, over-drink, over-eat, or take drugs?

3. We practice being in the present:
   When you "take your hands off your ears", and "open your eyes", guess what? It's just like it was a few moments ago...nothing went away and nothing changed. But this is also your first experience at being in the present moment, and at this point you are just watching. Breathe, relax, and allow the thoughts and feelings to come up and move through you as you bring your attention back to your breath.

When you practice being in the present moment, you begin

to allow other sensations to occur. Despite any desire to avoid or run, stay with it and feel each sensation arise. Something might come up as the sensation is moving through the body. Tears might come, you could begin laughing, or you might want to scream. These are natural expressions that help us release the intensity of the feelings. Allow it to happen. Remind yourself that you are releasing. Simply breathe through it and relax.

Too often we forget that we can choose our thoughts. Our thoughts do not choose us unless they come up as an habitual thought pattern. If you feel you cannot stop thinking about something that is bothering you, practice the skills that increase your ability to gather your attention and focus your energies so you can redirect them in a more positive way.

Evaluate the merit of each thought as it appears. Be an observer as if you were standing back and seeing it from the outside. What is the real purpose of this thought? What consequences will this thought bring about? How am I feeling (happy, sad, frustrated, unlovable, etc.)? Only from this perspective can you fairly evaluate the worthiness of each thought. This process helps you to train the mind to respond creatively, rather than react habitually. This is one of the keys to freedom.

4. We begin to shift to a state of calm and comfort:
   As you shift back to the present moment and begin to clearly see options and resources, your state of being begins to shift from unrest and/or fear to calm and comfort. The critical incidents in your life are not what disturb you as much as the state of helplessness you assign to yourself during these times. Though the crisis is a real condition, so is calm during crisis. This is achieved by practicing being in the present through using the rhythms of your breath and awareness.

   This shift to a state of calm and comfort is truly like reaching the crest of a hill. There is a kind of weightless experience where knowledge and experience begin to integrate as one. The mind and body blend to enjoy a balance. Feelings become empowered and invigorated with this collective transformation.

5. We are conscious of our freedom and ability to choose our actions:
   Through staying with the process of "climbing the emotional hill" you are developing skills designed to take back your power. Your personal power comes from the knowledge that you have free will and a conscious ability to positively affect your own life. The result is a sense of freedom. You are able to view painful, frustrating

situations in life with a series of "ah-ha" moments. You move from reactions to actions and see the results with a clarity that encourages you to continue practicing the process of shifting to the present moment so you can reproduce the results.

However overwhelming or "scary", emotions have an energy that must be expressed and released. Repressing, denying and avoiding your emotions prevent the release of that emotional energy. When there is crying, or being emotional, or having extreme feelings, there is energy being released. This is healthy and necessary. You may also cry when you are overwhelmed with joy or to release a past held tension or stuck emotional state.

Crying, laughing, and other natural expressions of emotion show that we already instinctively know to some extent what is healthy and what we need in order to move through our experiences in life. Teaching yourself to incorporate conscious breathing into this process will help form an automatic response to upsetting incidents.

There is a profound difference between being helpless and powerless. When you stop in your car at a red light you are powerless over when the light will change to green. If someone were to stop at the red light and feel helpless about it, you would recognize that their feeling had nothing to do with the traffic light, or anything else, other than a feeling they had assigned to themselves.

When you are confronted with an issue that you are powerless over, only what is associated with that one issue goes "on hold". Everything else continues. But when you allow yourself to feel helpless, EVERYTHING stops; every portion of your life begins to shut down around one singular incident.

By re-framing your relationship with yourself with the goal of creating contentment and satisfaction, you will see that others will treat you differently. When you complete the process of "climbing the emotional hill" you authentically elevate and lighten your mood. You see yourself, your life, and the world around you in a different way. When you see your circumstances in a new way, your circumstances will actually change, and what you are attracting in the world will change.

"Being happy" happens when you unburden yourself of your own "stuff". No one can do it for you or take the load from you; it is not dependent on external circumstances beyond what you allow. If your feelings have been hurt, remind yourself, only you can hurt your feelings by giving others power to do so.

Step three of climbing the emotional hill uses the word "practice". That term is used quite literally. At first, you have to make the process of being in the present moment a very conscious and deliberate act. Don't wait to apply it only in an emergency. Try it for the smallest things, and let the process grow and become a natural part of your experience of life. Create an experience of free will, calm, and awareness for yourself. Be ready for whatever life brings.

# Chapter 9 - treating yourself with kindness

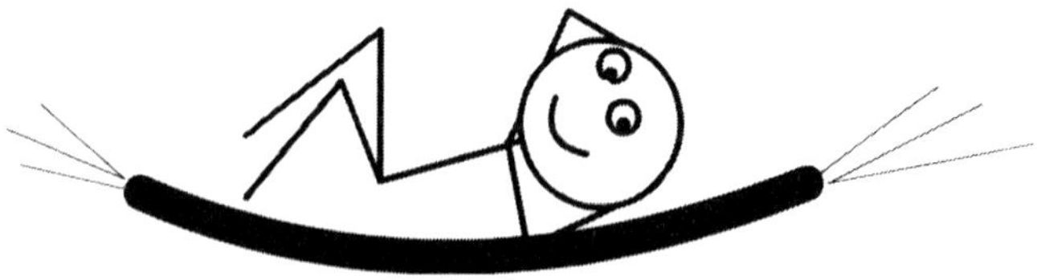

When you begin practicing self-awareness, you may become frustrated with your experience and with yourself. It is very easy, and common, to have a desire to change and make healthier choices but find that you are not yet able to do so. You will see how you judge, criticize, and beat yourself up, and then judge yourself for doing so and not being able to stop.

Remember, those thought patterns, beliefs, stands, habits and "buttons" did not form overnight. It will take time and conscious, repetitive practice to instill the newer, life-affirming thoughts, beliefs and behaviors. You would not expect a baby to learn to run five minutes after learning to crawl. Treating yourself with the same kindness, patience and encouragement that you would show that baby will make a huge impact on your progress in your journey to living life as a joyful being.

## AUTOBIOGRAPHY IN FIVE SHORT CHAPTERS

*by Portia Nelson*

I.

I walk down the street.
There is a deep hole in the sidewalk
I fall in.
I am lost...I am helpless.
It isn't my fault.
It takes me forever to find a way out.

II.

I walk down the same street.
There is a deep hole in the sidewalk.
I pretend I don't see it.
I fall in again.
I can't believe I am in the same place
but, it isn't my fault.
It still takes a long time to get out.

III.

I walk down the same street.
There is a deep hole in the sidewalk.
I see it is there.
I still fall in...it's a habit.

my eyes are open
I know where I am.
It is my fault.
I get out immediately.

IV.

I walk down the same street.
There is a deep hole in the sidewalk.
I walk around it.

V.

I walk down another street.

Treating yourself with kindness is not about self-compliments, or painting a picture of yourself in your mind without the "blemishes" or parts you perceive as unattractive. Your personality has a bright side and a dark side (that part of yourself that is capable of cruelty and destruction). You can choose which side to use to achieve balance and equanimity.

It's interesting to observe the affects and differences that occur when you react to situations using either the "bright" or the "dark" side. You may notice that you react using the "dark" side of your personality to respond to confrontations.

When you respond to a confrontation with the negative part of your personality (aggressiveness, intimidation, anger, etc.), the effects are immediate. You usually see an obvious and immediate result. When you respond to a confrontation with the positive part of your personality (kindness, patience, reason, understanding, etc.), the effects are much more subtle and not immediately apparent. Utilizing your positive personality traits produces more productive results. Yet human nature produces a desire for the immediate and obvious over the subtle and timely.

When you practice being kind to yourself and recognizing your ability to choose how you react, factor in that human desire for the more immediate solution (which tends to be the less productive path). Having patience with yourself is the first kindness you give yourself, and will guide your way to bringing other kindnesses into your life.

***You cannot be kind to others until***
***you are first kind to yourself***

Begin the process of being kind to yourself by:

**Bringing Awareness**

Become willing to open your eyes to new truths or realities and experience an awareness of new-found conditions or perspectives. Simply observe your self-talk. Do you speak kindly to yourself? Are you constantly negative or self-critical? As you let go of the illusions of negative self-image and perfection, you become willing to look at and own your mistakes and triumphs in an equal manner. Being truthful with yourself, knowing your limits, and respecting them frees you up to have more vital energy so you can be more creative and balanced in everything you do. Living in integrity with yourself allows you to be truly intimate with yourself and others.

**Recognizing That You Are Not Alone**

You live your life in various relationships. There are many interactions on many different levels. Just as no individual human being is "perfect", there are no "perfect" relationships. Yet, each relationship is perfect just as it is because it provides opportunities for self-awareness and growth. You can be kind one minute and cruel the next, or enjoy someone else's kindness or be a victim of their cruelty. By realizing that all people have negative and positive responses day to day, you can avoid being self-critical.

**Practicing Self-Care**

Taking care of yourself and taking charge of your life are the best ways to say you are worthwhile. They are personal acknowledgements of your self-worth, and they require no one else to validate you.

As you let go of the dependence on external circumstances to "make you happy" you are no longer tossed about in the waves of emotions. When you cultivate acceptance, gratitude and balance you begin the process of healing. By incorporating healthy habits such as exercise, adequate sleep, nourishing food, meditation and relaxation, you will begin to gain peace of mind and harmony.

**Healing the Numbness**

If you observe the people around you, many have experienced traumatic events in their life history. Trauma creates a numbness and resistance to new thoughts and establishes a pattern of thinking that leads you to believe that change is not possible. It is important to realize that you *have* these thoughts and emotions but are not *made of* these thoughts and emotions. They are just something you have carried along over time.

Traumatic experiences can take many forms and can cause the body and mind to be stuck in a frozen state. The body signals that it's not safe either inside yourself or outside in the world. You no longer trust yourself or others around you, no matter what the relationship may be. Your body feels like it is constantly fighting an existing enemy. Blood pressure rises, heart rate increases, stress hormones flood the body and it feels like the incident just happened. Physical movement, such as stretching, help ease the feelings of helplessness, fear, arousal, and numbness that may arise. Bringing awareness to this trauma-related biological condition is a kindness to yourself that can then increase a willingness to re-direct your attention as you bring mindfulness to your surroundings.

**Releasing Shame and Pain**

You've been conditioned by your parents and society to have wants and needs. It is rare in our culture to have been brought up to have peace of mind. You accumulate frustrations from wanting and needing that which artificially defines your worth. In the course of a lifetime these habits can range from simple shortcomings to serious detrimental behaviors. These inaccuracies begin to form the feeling that your insides do not match your outsides. Your kindness to yourself in this situation is to accept your unbalanced sense of guilt and shame, rather than moralizing and judging it.

Take a much less dramatic route. Visualize "the software of your mind". See your current situation as programming that has been haphazardly fixed, patched, and added to over time until no one is sure what the software was designed to originally accomplish.

You are the computer technician for the "software of your mind". You're not sure what button on the program does what, because over time everything has been relabeled and mislabeled. First you go in and try temporarily shutting down any functions that are not absolutely necessary. In the contemplative sense this would be the first step of meditation, in quieting the inner dialogue. In the corporate world, this would be having your secretary clearing your schedule, and filing away documents scattered on your desk.

Next, to fix the "software of your mind", you begin to trace back circuits from their buttons to the actions they create. As part of a meditative process this would be the breathing, as it oxygenates the body connecting and aligning all its parts. For the office executive this would be contacting various consultants for a conference.

And finally you would put your "software of the mind" back online, one function at a time. You deal with each function individually first, rather than turning the program on entirely in one quick move. The meditative example would be the yoga participant who moves each part of his body individually before attempting to take on a complex pose involving all the limbs. The corporate example would be auditing each spreadsheet before presenting a budget to the Board Members.

These examples may seem to stretch how you can be kind to yourself. Simplify the issues into their elements, and take on the challenges with each element rather than as a whole. You can then become aware of the conditions under which you operate. Then you can proceed with a calm mind...this is the greatest kindness of all to give yourself.

# Chapter 10 – mechanics of the mind

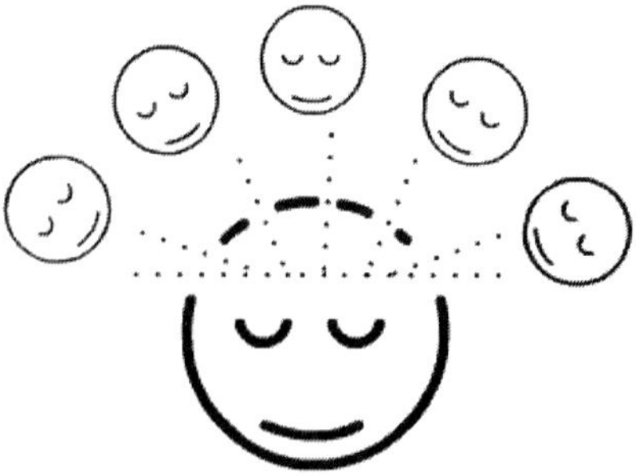

**"Nothing is more important than being able to choose the way we think – our feelings, aspirations, and desires; the way we view our world and ourselves. Mastery of the mind means that we can begin to reshape our life and character, rebuild relationships, thrive in the stress of daily living and become the kind of person we really want to be."**

- *Eknath Easwaran*

Thought and thinking requires the brain. Obvious as it is, taking the way the brain functions into deliberate consideration is a significant advantage when applying the studies and exercises of this manual. We have spoken about your thoughts, feelings, energy, breathing, and perceptions. These all join to work together in the brain.

We will leave most of the neurology to the men of medicine and present just some concepts about the brain that can provide you a more effective visualization of this amazing component of the body.

The Brain:

1. Weighs about 3 lbs
2. Uses 25% of the calories we consume
3. Uses 20% of the oxygen we breathe
4. Uses 25% of our blood flow
5. Contains cells, neurons, and the reactive synapses… billions of them!

So, again, it is obvious that when you have thoughts, feelings, perceptions, and speech there is some serious physiology going on! Combining your awareness of the physical aspect of your brain with your studies of your thoughts and emotions helps you to understand the brain responses that occur as you go through the process of mastering your thoughts, emotions and behaviors.

We are conscious of only a portion of our mental activity, and much of our thinking and feeling takes place totally outside of our awareness. As has been said before, our thinking process creates the "stories" about our life. These stories may include self-criticism and self-condemnation. Guilt and shame grow in us. We feel weak emotionally and physically. We often feel "not in control". The anonymous quote "No one can make me feel guilty without my consent" is so true. You unconsciously participate in "beating up" on yourself. As you might have noticed, it seems like you are either in collaboration or in confrontation with your mind.

You can learn to redirect your mind through breath work, introspection and visualization. As you gain strength through inner communication with yourself, this will aid you in increasing rather than decreasing your powers.

Often, human emotions, thoughts, and behavior are powered by four basic urges. These channels of energy arise from four primitive unconscious fountains, which are your desires for food, sex, sleep and self-preservation. Like a geyser, these fountains are not always active. When one channel is operating, the thought might have the force of being pulled by a hundred horses. The primitive fountain may also be dormant and it could have no power to make you act.

Though you cannot shut down the initial urges that come into your awareness from the four primitive fountains, you do have the capacity to decide how to redirect the energy. The simple recognition of compulsive thoughts that originate from one of these primal urges can begin the harnessing of its power and decrease its control over us. The practices of breathing techniques, meditation, visualization and physical movement will help you gain perspective to see changes that you can make and to gain the will power and skill to incorporate these changes in your daily life.

Without a discriminating mind, you will be at the mercy of compulsions, cravings and habits such as overeating, drug, alcohol or sex addiction, exhaustion, etc. Your energy will be wasted and contrary to your best interest. With a discriminating mind, you will be in harmony and free to choose your thoughts, words and actions to lead you to your greatest good.

**The "Command Control Center"**

Like a giant console of switches at a spaceship launch center, your brain is a complex bank of controls and switches. You can imagine what a small 7 year old would do on a school field trip to that spaceship launch center…he would start flipping every switch he could! And so do you sometimes...you just begin reacting by "flipping switches". In the example, the scientist would realize what our small boy was doing and would be hard pressed to undo the chaos. In your own life, when you flip switches haphazardly, it is near impossible to retrace your feelings and actions in an attempt to understand your responses and reactions.

In crisis mode, the scientist would not act like a seven year old and just start flipping switches. He would use his knowledge to make a choice in which switches to flip. You could use another example, replacing the scientist with someone who repeats the same actions over and over as part of his job. This worker automatically repeats the same actions out of habit. And so do some of us, always reacting with the same emotion to everything.

The point here is not to identify the "correct" combinations of switches in your brain. The idea is to be aware that the brain is always flipping switches. Whether you take control or not, the brain will always seek to resolve a contradiction in your thinking. It is your awareness of this behavior and your efforts to deliberately focus your thinking that will guide your personal Command Control Center to flip switches in a beneficial, useful way.

**Taking Care of the Brain**

The brain is a living organ. It requires nutrients, oxygen, water, and positive stimulation. It can be injured, and it can become diseased. You can poison your brain in so many ways, with just a few encounters with dangerous substances (drugs, chemicals, etc), or repeated contact with potentially unhealthy substances (alcohol, tobacco). You can injure the brain through accidents and dangerous activities.

There is a saying that "your cup is full to overflowing, you cannot take one more thing in until you dump something out". Nutrition, circulation, digestion, elimination, adequate sleep, relaxation, and types of meditation are all aspects of "emptying your cup to make room for more". Give your brain time to clear out the cobwebs, creating space for new possibilities.

# Chapter 11 – integrity with yourself

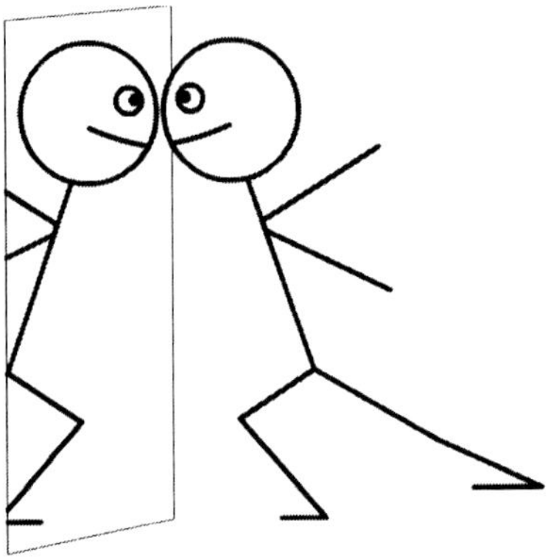

**"This above all: to thine own self be true,**

**And it must follow, as the night the day,**

**Thou canst not then be false to any man."**

\- *William Shakespeare*

Many of us are familiar with the words "To thine own self be true" from William Shakespeare's *Hamlet*, but we may not be as familiar with the rest of that sentence. In it, Shakespeare is telling us that when we have integrity with ourselves by being true to ourselves we will then, by default, have integrity with others and the world around us. Once again, our experience of life is completely based on how we are with ourselves.

Integrity with yourself is the matching of your "insides" with your "outsides". When "how we are" and "who we are" in the world is not the same as "how we are" and "who we are" inside, there is inner conflict and contradiction.

When what we want for our life and how we want to live our life takes a back seat to living based on who we think we have to be in the world and what others expect from us, we are out of integrity with ourselves and live a life filled with stress and emotional pain.

To cope with this ongoing stress and emotional pain we deny, repress, suppress, and avoid through addictions and addictive behaviors. We lash out at those around us, and we stay "stuck" in reactive mode. Physical illness and chronic health conditions may even result from the physiological impact of the ongoing stress.

Having the courage to acknowledge those conflicts and contradictions and deciding that your relationship with yourself is important enough to make it your priority are steps on the path toward being in integrity with yourself. Then, when you are in integrity with yourself, you can begin living in integrity with the world around you.

How authentic are you? How well do your insides match your outsides? Make a list of areas of your life where things don't match up. Then, look at each area and begin to question your intent behind the choices you made. What is your pay-off for living inauthentically? We always have a reason, and it is usually a good one...even a big one. Sometimes it even feels like "life or death".

**Example**: *You come from a family of doctors or lawyers or police officers or farmers. Whatever the profession, it runs in your family and runs in your blood. It is the profession the family expected you to pursue, and it is the profession you pursued. But it was not who you wanted to be. Instead of being an architect, you wanted to be a musician. Instead of managing one of the family's chain of retail stores, you wanted to explore the world. You go to work each day, and may even find some enjoyment or satisfaction from your work. Yet, there is still that longing...that little voice calling to you and reminding you that this life is just not "you". You still have the dream, but maybe it hurts too much to think of it every day, so you do things to avoid hearing that voice. You drink, you watch hours of television, or you may even work extra hours at the job you don't like just to keep busy and distracted.*

Using the example above, let's examine this situation a little further. You chose to deny your dream profession or lifestyle for the sake of the family. Why? Out of love, sure, but maybe also out of a sense of belonging, a sense of duty or obligation, or a sense of identity. Maybe while growing up you were told, either directly or indirectly, that "this is who we are when we are a member of this family". Makes sense...but there is still more to uncover.

We've begun to look at the reasons why you originally made the choice to pursue the family profession, but what are the reasons that keep you from making a different choice now? What do you believe will happen if you give up the family business or profession? What would the consequences be?

Maybe there is fear of abandonment...fear of no longer belonging...fear of being disowned...fear of being ridiculed...fear of failing out there on your own...or fear of breaking the rules. These are all very powerful potential "consequences" of choosing "you" over the family. These are all very valid reasons for the choice you made. There is no judgment here, and no reason to judge yourself for making this choice. As always, this process is simply about awareness.

Now, ask yourself: are the possible consequences what *really* would happen, based on the individuals involved, or are the consequences what the scared child in you believes will happen?

Then, regardless of whether it is a "real" or "perceived" consequence, ask yourself: are your personal integrity, authenticity, peace, passion, joy, and dreams worth compromising or giving up in order to avoid those consequences?

At the moment, your answer might be "yes". Maybe your answer would still be "yes" one year, five years, or fifty years from now. That is ok. Because now you know what your motivations are. Now you can see what your priorities are. Now you have some self-awareness around this issue. And that self-awareness opens a door to new possibilities for you. When you are ready, *if* you are ready, you can begin to take steps to move towards the life you truly want to live.

When we shine a spotlight on our degree of integrity with ourselves, we often find many areas where we are out of balance. Some of these areas may be "major", such as in the example above, but others are minor little things that occur every day.

You are not stuck forever with a fixed set of feelings and life conditions. Where are your actions genuine and where are they a matter of convenience or perceived requirement? Where are your choices a part of your goals, and where are they just a mandatory action to "survive"? What do you tell yourself you will do, and what do you actually do?

Not every act required by your workplace or culture can be considered a genuine expression of your true feelings. Not every diplomatic comment made to spare someone's feelings will be actually an honest expression. Integrity with yourself can be found in the knowledge that these conditions and contrasts exist in you. Once you identify them, you can then choose where and how to shift your thinking to become as authentic as possible.

Moving towards being in integrity with yourself is the beginning of reacquiring your power. A key element of gaining back personal power is the introduction of new possibilities. Seeing where you may be out of integrity with yourself and examining your reasons "why" allows you to truly see what your choices and motivations were in the past and what they are in the present moment. From this information comes your power.

When you examine your life and identify your goals and dreams, then compare them to your present conditions, you begin to align your capabilities with your possibilities. Your possibilities are open wider than you ever imagined when you align them with your capabilities. Your capabilities can take you farther then you've ever thought, if you will just allow your "raw" desires to surface.

Remember those thoughts you had as a child about who you could become and what you would do? You desired it! You had a belief about all the possibilities in your future! You expected it could happen, and in your imagination you saw it actually happen! Anything CAN happen…you can create any possibility if these things are in place: DESIRE, BELIEF, and EXPECTATION.

As you grew, the external pressures overcame all these free independent desires and beliefs. You conformed to all the patterns of the world and lost sight of your specific purpose - your unique contribution. You became a human doing rather than a human being. Your insides and outsides stopped matching. You began to wear "masks" and presented yourself to the world in the way the world expected of you. You conformed to the world's patterns.

What are the first steps for achieving integrity with yourself? You are a human being…just be! You want to be in a place where you can focus and be receptive to your own thoughts. As always, making your physical self still, relaxed, and quiet is to your best advantage.

Sit quietly, breathe, acknowledge any thoughts or distractions, and let them go to get to the Neutral Mind. Wait expectantly for the voice within...your voice…your truth…your integrity.

From the "inside-out" you will begin to speak your truth and take actions with integrity. Eventually you will achieve your highest potential, feel the warmth of personal fulfillment and live life to the fullest.

Getting to know yourself with a fair and balanced perspective of your inner and outer conditions is the key. Examining your choices and motivations and admitting that you have a "bright" side and "dark" side to your perceptions, actions and reactions gives you the realistic basis to look closely at the emotional balances in your life and achieve a level of integrity and authenticity.

Feeling guilt, resentment, and regret robs you of your power. Your loss of personal power leaves you disconnected from your "self" and more likely to live according to what is outside of your "self" – the world around you and the expectations of that world. From that position, you are even more likely to make choices that are inauthentic and out of integrity with yourself...and the vicious cycles continue.

Confronting the mismatches of your outsides and your insides and choosing to shift your thoughts and actions in a way that leaves you feeling balanced and honest with yourself…*this* is finding integrity with yourself.

# Chapter 12 – introspection

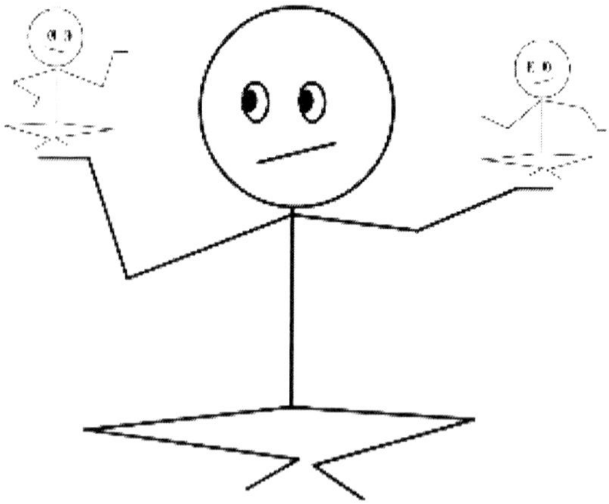

We know now that we can take more control over our lives by looking internally at what is really going on. When we observe, examine, and shift our primary thinking habits including beliefs, stands, and "buttons" we gain self-awareness, empowerment, and peace of mind. Beginning or expanding a practice of introspection and meditation can greatly aid us in this process.

Remember, meditation is simply getting to know yourself on a deeper level. We have often given our power away by letting everyone else tell us what "our truth" is. Meditation is an enjoyable and energizing experience you can use to train and calm the mind. A healthy body and mind are the benefits of skills you learn in meditation and introspection.

The terms introspection and meditation appear to be on

opposite sides of the cultural scale, one associated with western thought and the other eastern. But each has almost identical components and similar results for those who implement the practice. Each requires an active, inward look at yourself in search of your "truth".

The classic benefits associated with both introspection and meditation are:

1. Creating a calming effect, a release of tension
2. Creating an environment to find resolution
3. Cultivating a more kind or understanding perspective
4. Achieving a healthier lifestyle
5. Increasing energy and the ability to focus

You will be taught the steps to begin introspection later in this chapter. For now, let's assume you are capable of introspection or meditation, and look at the processes and results from a different angle. During introspection you will learn to let go of unnecessary thoughts and unneeded distractions and eliminate or lessen sensations. These external distractions are similar to radio signal interference, or "static". The source of this "static" is often an external physical source. In a relaxed state you can learn to moderate your sensations and reactions to the static.

Introspection and meditation are not emotional diversions. They are not only religious activities. They are not really even intellectual tactics. Even a corporate executive who needs to focus on a specific problem or issue by looking for a "gut" feeling will choose to separate himself from distractions in order to find an answer within. This same executive would certainly not surround himself with noise and activity while in contemplation. He would shut his office door, instruct his secretary to hold his calls, and find a comfortable place to sit.

And so the technique begins with the physical…breathing. Your mind starts to wander through this breathing process...to the past, to the future, to a sound, to a physical feeling, etc. Immediately the pattern of the breath begins to break. The breathing quickens and becomes slightly more laborious. This shows you how the breath and thinking are linked. Your body is also reacting to physical sensations (an ache, a pain, room temperature, etc.) Meditation often provides you with insulations from these distractions.

By bringing your awareness back to your breathing you also calm your mind and body. As in our prior example, the executive can now resolve a problem more effectively and make decisions from a clearer perspective. You see how breath connects the mind and body. You see how it is not the external event itself but your own thoughts and perception about the external event that affects your breathing, attention, and emotions.

You do not have to wait for a problem to solve in order to practice introspection and meditation. It is perhaps even better to practice without the distraction of an immediate issue, so that the skill can become automatic.

Introspection is the stripping away of distractions so that you are left with what truly belongs to you. You are simply adjusting the tuner on your mental radio so that the extra signals (sensations) do not add static to your personal radio station (your mind).

How do you create introspection? How do you begin to meditate?

1. **Environment** – Find a quiet place where you will not be disturbed. Sit in a comfortable physical position, whether it be in your favorite recliner chair or sitting cross-legged on a comfortable surface. You can visualize being in your favorite safe, comfortable environment (read the chapter on visualization for more information).

2. **Breathe** – Begin by conscientiously taking control of your breathing. Use an even, full "three-part-breath" which moves air from the lower diaphragm all the way through the upper portion of the clavicle. Slowly allow the breath to become even, smooth and finally automatic.

3. **Filter Out** – Allow each distracting thought to enter your mind - do not resist it. You can acknowledge it and bring your attention back to the breath as you let it go.

4. **Accept the Guest** – As the distractions subside, an

individual thought may come to the surface that you will chose to consider. Follow the thought and you may find one of two things will happen: either there will be no particularly significant thoughts and you will experience a feeling of restful peace and welcome waking sleep; or an individual thought will come to the surface that you will judge as important to consider. Try to allow that thought to play itself out without guiding its beginning or its conclusion.

It's important to note that when you begin introspection, the thought or issue of importance that surfaces may not be the same as your original intent for the session. If this happens, you may want to consider that resolution of this unanticipated issue and/or thought is actually necessary first in order to effectively deal with the issue that you originally considered your first priority.

5. **Complete the Circle** – Begin the process of winding down to the end of your session. Take your breathing back to a conscious "three-part-breath", and then let it even out to a smooth, easy rhythm. Occasionally return to the "three-part-breath" in order to maintain your attention to the breath; then let it once again return to an automatic even rhythm and your enjoyable vision. This last phase can be repeated for hours or minutes. You may even with to

conclude your session by lying down on your back with arms, legs, feet, hands, and head all in a neutral relaxed pose.

Meditation and introspection are not just thinking about something, like mindful breathing is not just taking deep breaths. You are conditioning your automatic response system. Learn the process at your own pace; your level of mastery will increase with time. If you are not ready to take 15 to 20 minutes to devote to a introspection and/or meditation session, you can still receive benefits during the course of your day by remembering to stay present and non-judgmental. Instead of looking at your watch, take a few moments to look within yourself.

# Chapter 13 – visualization

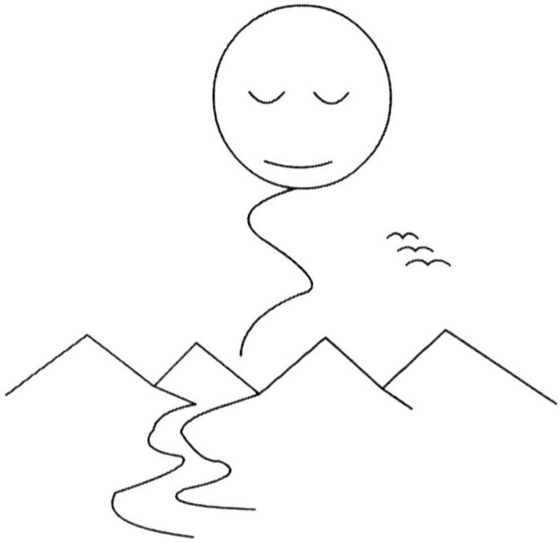

With visualizations we focus on achieving a desired result, bringing the best part of our talents forward to aid us in our efforts. The term is very literal, because in fact we create a vision for our intentions and the actions that will bring those intentions to reality. We actually visualize all of the time. We "see" the refrigerator before we get off the couch to go retrieve a snack, and we assemble the makings for our sandwich in our minds before we actually put it together on a plate.

Unfortunately we also visualize less ordinary and less positive events...for example, in the fine details of our imaginations we see the boss coming into our office to scold us for coming in late to work! We use the same process and amount of effort whether we visualize positive or negative outcomes. It is with the strength of your intent that you can choose what you would like to see.

While visualizing is traditionally used as a tool for achieving goals, there are many other benefits:

1. You look more closely at what it is you truly want and begin to see the differences between wants, needs, desires, and dreams.

2. Your thoughts and goals learn to merge into organized actions.

3. Your ability to concentrate increases in time and intensity.

4. A collection of possibilities for your life begins to build, providing the foundations to imagine even more possibilities.

5. You increase your ability to differentiate between a coherent vision and illogical "imaginings".

6. With growing possibilities, clear ideas, and a better grasp of your real goals, confidence grows within you and you are more consistently relaxed and rested.

Visualizations are not just making a snapshot in your mind of that final moment when "you cross the finish line, winning the big race". Visualizations are a series of mental images that build and connect to each other in the same ways a successful victory would be achieved. Even in the course of your daily life, this process helps to organize your thinking and provide clarity to your goals. It forms your thinking and projections around the elements of success in order to create that final result built from all those smaller parts.

**Example:** *<u>The Runner</u> - The track and field competitor doesn't just visualize his final victorious stride across the finish line. He sees himself in his mental picture at a time months before, stretching, lifting weights, conditioning. He sees himself practicing his start in the runner's blocks. He feels himself running faster and faster; faster than he has ever run before. He feels all the air he needs coming easily into his lungs, all of his muscles flexing as if they will never tire. He finally visualizes himself running through a crowd passing other runners one by one, until he sees no one in front of him. Visualizations can include inspirations. He can see his father and himself a decade before, with his father encouraging him to run faster through their lawn.*

**Example:** <u>*Employee Late to Work*</u> – *The employee, knowing his boss will soon be in his office to scold him for being late to work, can visualize the best outcome possible. He can see the boss come in, and rather than wait for the boss to speak, he sees himself standing, greeting the boss and beginning the conversation about his late start. He can in his imagination hear himself discuss it with his boss without excuses, and with a straightforward amends instead of an insincere apology. He visualizes his boss being receptive, accepting that the issue is resolved. With this positive visualization of a potentially negative situation, the employee will project an entirely different presence to the boss in the real encounter yet to occur. The boss will see someone honest, confident, and competent to handle difficult situations, instead of someone fearful, hesitant, and unsure what to say.*

**Example:** <u>*The Busy Manager (Visualize It Backwards)*</u> – *The Manager has a complex task to complete that will require the cooperation of her entire staff. She has received her assignment, but has never attempted a similar project before. So she visualizes it backwards! She sees the final presentation in her mind, assembling all the segments of the event. In her mind she assigns each segment to a particular staff member. Her imagination pictures each individual person and develops a plan for how to prepare that staffer with both information and encouragement. One at a time she visualizes placing* *resources each staff member will need on their desks. It does not matter if they will need a big projection screen or 100 feet of network cord, the Manager "sees" it piled around the staff member's desk! She creates an image of her staff as an orchestra, each performing on a different instrument and playing together. Finally (and this applies to all the above examples) she will visualize "impeccable intent". Her visualization becomes not a picture in her mind but a feeling she allows to radiate through her body. She cultivates in her being a force of will...a strong resolve...an impeccable intent to accomplish her goal using only positive means and absolute certainty of outcome.*

You have experienced this strength of will and intent, normally when you are extremely happy and confident or extremely angry. But your goal in visualization is to make positive visualizations a part of your natural rhythms; an automatic part of your recognition of events and the solution process. As we practice visualization in a purposeful manner, there is a high probability you will begin to call upon it without even consciously creating a vision.

OK, Let's Visualize!

1. **Get Started** – let's practice with all the conditions in our favor...comfortable chair, quiet room, closed eyes. Start

breathing our "three-part-breath" all the way from the diaphragm to the collar bone, deep even and full. Now calm the breath to even soft rhythms.

2. **Start Simple** – With your eyes closed, see if you can make a picture of a tree in your mind. Make it very specific, with exact shape, branches and leaves. Now change the color of the leaves to fall colors, and then no leaves at all for the winter.

3. **Move Objects** – Visualize coins in your pocket. See yourself pull the coins out and spread them in front of you. Stack the coins in separate piles, pennies, nickels, dimes, etc. Now pickup a stack of coins and put it behind you where you cannot see it, keep it up until there are no stacks in your view.

4. **People** – Visualize someone you know. Be careful, with people you know you tend to visualize too quickly what is already familiar, so try to see all the details about that person you can recall. Change their facial expression; see them smile in your mind's view. See them yawn.

5. **Step In / Step Out** – Visualize your friend, and now step into the scene you have created. In your mind's eye pull

back and see both you and your friend in the same "scene".

6. **Move** – While you relax in your chair with your eyes closed, keep your hands to your side and your head straight ahead. Now without moving, visualize raising and lowering your arm. Finally visualize not only turning your head to the side, but see what you would see if you were looking in that direction.

Whew! Hard work? What did it accomplish? It is a routine that exercises a portion of your brain most of us rarely use or use only to a small fraction of our potential. When you learn to combine the imagination, the spatial concept part of your brain, with the logical and memory portions of the brain, a powerful chemistry of visualization begins to brew. The span of what you can logically conceive of is expanded by your imagination; and your expanded capability for logic stimulates your imagination! Both merge to form possibilities for your life, and visualization creates a positive path to achieve your true goals.

# Chapter 14 – a few good moves

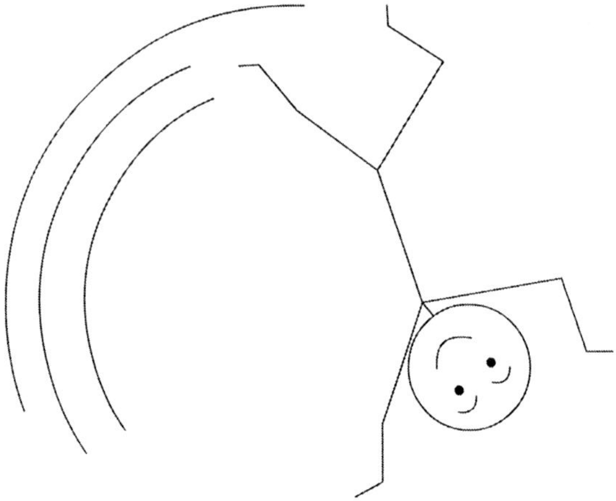

Just as your body responds to your thoughts, your thoughts respond to your body! Introducing a routine of motion and movement into your daily life, to whatever degree you are physically able to do so, provides a benefit to your physical brain as well as to your mind. When mind and body utilize each other in actions, "simultaneous communication" is formed. The mind and body witness each other and a balanced centering is created. These movements can be traditional (basketball, golf, tennis) or they can be classical (yoga, tai chi, pilates). In addition, movements for well-being can be simply spontaneous and for fun!

Whatever the case, combining breath, mind, and motion serve to rejuvenate all your body's systems. Your muscular, skeletal, circulatory, digestive, endocrine, evacuation, and immune systems all respond to a routine of movement.

With movement a release is experienced. Tension dissipates, energy is produced, concentration becomes easier, and a state of calm and confidence can result.

Balancing, twisting, stretching, and exerting are things you can learn to do better and better with practice. There is unlimited potential for your body and mind to excel in balanced poses or changing motions. Then, below the surface of all that is visible, are the neurons firing signals in your brain, the nerves transmitting electronic micro-bits of energy, oxygen molecules flowing throughout the body to be consumed, gathered, and consumed again.

Of all the lessons in your *Joyful Being* guide that discuss emotions, perspective, perception, and awareness, let's never forget that wherever you take these skills for living, your body must always be there too to contribute as well as benefit. Your body is not just a suitcase that holds everything inside. Your thoughts and feelings merge seamlessly with your body. The more you engage them together in concert, the better all of them work for you.

You begin to experience this as giving a valuable gift to yourself and see fun and activity as an essential part of your living life as a *joyful being*.

# Chapter 15 - joyful being

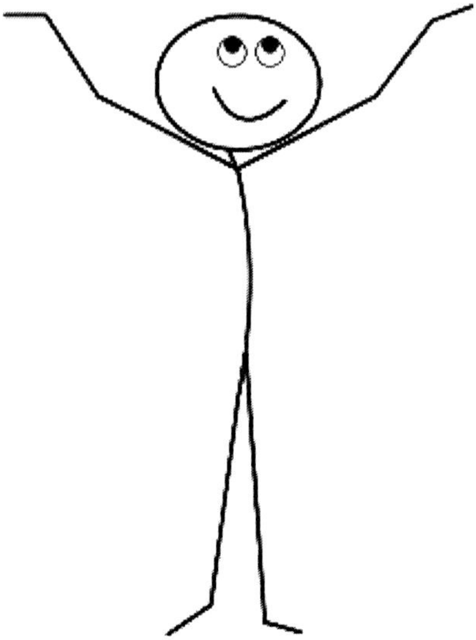

You get a call on your telephone. It's the local radio station calling to say you are on the air, and if you answer their quiz question of the day, you will win a great prize. The DJ asks, "What color was George Washington's white horse?" You answer "white!" And you win. Immediately you want to know three things: What is the prize? What is it worth? And how do I get it?

Of all the chapters in this book, a chapter specifically suggesting that you can experience "living life as a joyful being" is the one where answers to these three questions will be sought. All the philosophy, conjecture, and science come in second place to the possibility that you can live a happy, content, and serene life.

## *What is it, what's it worth, how do I get it?*

**What is it?**

"Joyful Being" is a spontaneous moment when the physical, mental, and emotional become one, fused together in a very physiological way. It is not your imagination projecting with such a desire to be peaceful that you force yourself to believe you are. It is a truly living state where body, mind, and heart share a single consciousness; where you not only feel peace, but you ***are*** peace.

Your self-love is not just a gesture to yourself in any individual moment, but a continuous action. Your own joyful being is something you can take ownership of, cultivate and allow to grow. It is an expression of your true, authentic nature. Every human seeks to be a joyful being because his or her inner-most thoughts recall this state of being from their earliest memories as an infant. As you were domesticated by your histories and the stories others have had you believe, you lost your way and you lost the means to restore that capacity that each of us has within us to become a joyful being.

**What is it worth?**

Living life as a joyful being provides you with many gifts:

- A new sense of who you are
- Clarity of your own self-image and the world around you
- An expanded capacity to love yourself

- A sense of satisfaction and appreciation for the present
- The absence of obsession with resentments of the past and fear of the future
- A life force that allows you to make healthy choices and goals that provide you with positive results
- The desire and power to live your life as a self-creative being instead of as a self-destructive one
- Complete freedom to live as your true self with an unobstructed view of your happiness

**How do I get it?**

You resolve to be in and breathe fully into the present moment. In other words, you make a conscious decision (resolve) to settle the body (with breath) and see the world around you with objectivity (balance) so that your perceptions and perspectives come from real (the present) moments of your experience. With this as the foundation, your first sensation is freedom. From freedom comes empowerment; and from empowerment comes knowledge. From knowledge comes peace. From peace comes joy.

Resolve is necessary because your first efforts result in just that…*efforts*. You need dedication of purpose to make that conscious decision to continually focus on doing the work until you experience the rewards. Breathing and awareness of your body is a necessary part of the process, because living as a joyful being includes the physical state of being as well. Finally, objectivity and balance provide fresh, healthy perspectives and the inner integrity to give your joyful being a home for it to live. It is the "being" part of your joy.

## *So Where Do I Go From Here?*

Through each of the previous chapters of this book, we have examined the many ways that we hold ourselves back and limit ourselves with our thoughts, beliefs, and stories from the past. If you are reading this page, then hopefully you have also read at least some of what has come before it. You now realize there is no "quick fix" or "miracle pill" that will make it all better in five minutes. As you read each chapter, you may have begun recognizing areas where the ideas in this book relate to your life. You may even have begun to consider new perspectives. Now, the fun begins.

From the time you were born, you have been playing this game called "living". However, if you were like most of us, you were never taught the *true* rules...the ones that say YOU get to determine your beliefs, your identity, your story, and the script for the movie of your life. While many others have provided input (whether you wanted it or not!), only *you* have final edit and approval for the script.

As you read this book, you began to learn the REAL rules for this game. Now, *you* get to decide how you want to play. You get to decide how much of this "work" you want to do, how quickly you want to do this "work", and how much you want it to *feel* like "work". Have fun! Be gentle and loving with yourself. Laugh at yourself and your "human-ness" along the way. You are not alone; it is a condition we all suffer from. Be "in the moment", if only for one moment each day. Walk a few steps backwards so you can see how easy it is to change your perspective. Give yourself permission to be...to be who you are, and who you have been, all along...authentically, deep inside...a magnificent, incredible, *Joyful Being*!

***Let the games begin!***

# About the Author

Joy Jangdhari is a researcher and the author of "Living Life As A Joyful Being: be ready for whatever life brings! Her ground-breaking workshop "Technology for your Psychology" provides Continuing Education credits for Professional and Personal development. Ms. Jangdhari has received great reviews in recognition of her efforts to communicate the behavioral aspects of the mind-body connection and how it affects us all. Ms. Jangdhari is recommended by Doctors, Counselors, Therapists, Teachers & Entrepreneurs!

Joy Jangdhari President- Operation Dare To Care LLC

CEO- Joy Events LLC

TV producer and host of two educational, inspirational & motivational Television Talk Shows in New York City.

Ms. Jangdhari also uses these concepts in her own life.

www.JoyJangdhari.com

# Notes